The Staff and the Serpent

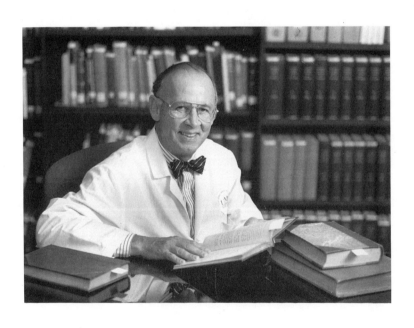

THE STAFF AND THE SERPENT

Pertinent and Impertinent Observations on the World of Medicine

Allen B. Weisse, M.D.

Southern Illinois University Press
Carbondale and Edwardsville

Copyright © 1998 by the Board of Trustees,
Southern Illinois University
All rights reserved
Printed in the United States of America
01 00 99 98   4 3 2 1

Library of Congress Cataloging-in-Publication Data

Weisse, Allen B.
The staff and the serpent : pertinent and impertinent observations on the world of medicine / Allen B. Weisse.
        p. cm.
Includes index.
1. Medicine—Philosophy. 2. Medicine—Anecdotes. I. Title.
[DNLM: 1. Medicine—essays. W 9 W432s 1998]
R723.W39   1998
610—dc21
DNLM/DLC
for Library of Congress
ISBN 0-8093-2149-1 (alk. paper)
97-5480
CIP

The paper used in this publication meets the minimum requirements of American National Standard for Information Sciences—Permanence of Paper for Printed Library Materials, ANSI Z39.48-1984. ⊚

To Laura

Contents

A Note on the Title xi

Preface xiii

Acknowledgments xv

1
Greetings 1

2
Betrayal 18

3
The Vanishing Male 26

4
Pneumocystis and Me: The Small Joys and Great Satisfactions of Medical Sleuthing 29

5
Tuberculosis: Why "The White Plague"? (Another Detective Story) 37

6
Say It Isn't "No": The Power of Positive Thinking in the Publication of Medical Research 45

7
Beyond the Bench: A Vote for Clinical Research 50

8
Mostly about Books—and Medicine 54

9
Confessions of Creeping Obsolescence 60

10
Man's Best Friend 64

11
"Non-Cognitive" Comes Home to Roost 69

12
Bats in the Belfry or Bugs in the Belly? Helicobacter and the Resurrection of Johannes Fibiger 73

13
Whither Our Children? 86

14
A Sin for Saint William? 92

15
In the Service of the IRS 97

16
What's in a Name? 103

17
PC: Politically Correct or Potentially Corrupting? 107

18
SI Units: Wrong for the Right Reasons 112

19
The Long and the Short and the Rest of It 118

20
On Chinese Restaurants, Prolapsing Heart Valves, and Other Medical Conundrums   122

21
So, You Want to Be a Doctor?   129

22
While the Getting's Good   137

Index   145

A Note on the Title

AESCULAPIUS, THE Graeco-Roman god of medicine, was always depicted as leaning upon a staff entwined by a single serpent. It is this serpent-staff caduceus motif that validly represents the symbol of medicine rather than the two-snake winged staff that has been adopted by organizations such as the U.S. Army Medical Corps and others. The latter is the symbol of Hermes, the Greek messenger god (Mercury to the Romans).

The symbolism of the serpent and the staff in the healing art predates even the Greek and Roman civilizations. The snake, often representative of death or evil, also attained meaning in terms of fertility and immortality, perhaps because of its ability to shed its skin and thereby seemingly assume a second life. This quality of regeneration undoubtedly led to the snake being looked upon as a symbol of healing as well.

Preface

WHAT IS THE connection between a parasite found in the abdomen of a South American rodent and the AIDS epidemic? With the resurgence of tuberculosis, what have been our past conceptions and misconceptions about this other dreaded disease?

What might Chinese restaurants and rubber galoshes have in common? Can a worm actually cause cancer? (The Nobel Prize committee was obviously convinced of this some years back.) Why are we so negative about negative research, the kind that shows that something just is not so?

How do we choose our medical students—and what can you do to improve your chances of being among them? What is the darker side of some of those senior scientists entrusted with training our future medical investigators? Can today's doctors ever manage to keep up with new developments? If not, when should they give up, and how?

These are a few of the questions I have attempted to answer after a lifelong study of medicine and over three decades as a practitioner, teacher, and researcher. A number of essays that have evolved from this quest deal with topics that are obviously of great social, economic, and public health importance, while others deal with questions of a more frivolous nature (some might label them much-ado-about-nothing). However, whether serious or lighthearted, I have found each essay's subject matter irresistible in one way or another.

Those with a professional scientific background might be drawn to certain pieces while the general reader might find others more compelling. My hope is that all these observations—pertinent and impertinent alike—will be accessible to most readers and judged as equally informative and fascinating as they were to the author in the process of composing them.

Acknowledgments

SOME OF THE essays are appearing in print for the first time; others have been previously published, most often in shorter form, some under a different title. Most articles were previously published in *Hospital Practice*. These articles are "Pneumocystis and Me: The Small Joys and Great Satisfactions of Medical Sleuthing"; "Say It Isn't 'No': The Power of Positive Thinking in the Publication of Medical Research"; "Beyond the Bench: A Vote for Clinical Research"; "Mostly about Books—and Medicine" (originally published as "Books Doctors Read"); "Confessions of Creeping Obsolescence"; "Man's Best Friend"; " 'Non-Cognitive' Comes Home to Roost"; "Bats in the Belfry or Bugs in the Belly?: Helicobacter and the Resurrection of Johannes Fibiger" (originally published as "Barry Marshall and the Resurrection of Johannes Fibiger"); "Whither Our Children?"; "In the Service of the IRS"; "SI Units: Wrong for the Right Reasons"; "The Long and the Short and the Rest of It"; "On Chinese Restaurants, Prolapsing Heart Valves, and Other Medical Conundrums"; and "While the Getting's Good." Initially it was David W. Fisher who encouraged me to contribute to *Hospital Practice*; more recently Lee Powers, the current executive editor, has proved to be an equally gracious sponsor. My thanks to them and to *Hospital Practice* for granting permission to reprint these pieces in their present form.

Similar thanks must be extended to Dr. Richard L. Landau and *Perspectives in Biology and Medicine* for providing another forum for my work and granting permission to reproduce it. "The Vanishing Male"; "PC: Politically Correct or Potentially Corrupting?"; "What's in a Name?"; "Tuberculosis: Why 'The White Plague'? (Another Detective Story)" (originally published as "Tuberculosis: Why 'The White Plague'?"); were all previously published in *Perspectives in Biology and Medicine*, © 1988, 1994, 1995, 1996 by the University of Chicago. All rights reserved. "A Sin for Saint William?" published as "Osler, Aging and the Late Twentieth Century," is reprinted by permission of the publisher from *The Journal of Chronic Diseases*, vol. 30, pp. 473–75. Copyright 1977 by Elsevier Science Inc.

To all the patients, colleagues, students, house staff, friends, and family who stimulated me to write these essays—and they are too numerous to mention—I will remain eternally grateful as well.

The Staff and the Serpent

1

Greetings

ONE OF THE three panel members asked the applicant, "Would you mind explaining to us what it was that led you to apply again for admission to this medical school after having been turned down twice in the past?"

The young man replied, "It's true that I have been rejected by this school on two previous occasions, but each time I was informed by members of the Admissions Committee that I was well qualified and that they saw no reason why I should not make a good physician if accepted to your school. In view of their remarks, I felt that if I just kept coming back often enough, I just might work up a favorable majority on the committee and have my application approved."

The interviewing psychiatrist smiled; the surgeon frowned; the internist maintained a passive exterior. On that dismal day in 1953, I was going down for the third time in my unsuccessful attempts to obtain a place in the entering freshman medical school class of my alma mater, New York University. Before "submerging," however, I could not resist the opportunity of tweaking the bureaucratic noses of the experts who were making life so difficult for me. At that moment I had little expectation of ever becoming a doctor, let alone chairman of another medical school's admissions committee twenty years later.

My pathway into medicine was, indeed, long and circuitous. Originally destined to study law, I had switched to medicine after the experience of undergoing some minor surgery during my early high school years in New York City. The hospital atmosphere intrigued me, and I began reading books about the medical world, all of which strengthened my desire to become part of it. Only in later years was I to realize how ill-advised I had been in making many of the initial choices that would affect my joining the medical establishment.

My first mistake was my choice of college. Following my graduation from New York City's George Washington High School in 1946, I headed that fall to the University Heights campus of New York University in the Bronx. Although sold off some decades ago for financial reasons and now a community college of dubious academic standing, the Heights at that time was the "jewel in the crown" of New York University, the rest of its sprawling, mammoth operation confined to the streets of Greenwich Village surrounding Washington Square in lower Manhattan.

Roughly half of the Heights campus consisted of a highly respected school of engineering, some of whose departments were considered among the best in the country. The other half, the University College of Arts and Science, catered to the nonengineering students and was also felt to have a high academic standing, although not quite in league with a Harvard or Yale. Except for a half dozen women in the engineering school, the campus was an all male one with a total of less than four thousand students in all four years.

Physically, the campus deserved the appellation "jewel." Bounded on the east by bustling University Avenue, it immediately presented a pronounced rise in ground level, and the mounting of several flights of steps led one to a campus totally isolated from the hurly-burly of the surrounding city. In spring, especially, the blooming magnolias along the steps leading to the campus proper announced the entering of a different world and to this day evoke a potent memory of the place. On the westernmost perimeter of the campus, along the heights of the palisades overlooking the Harlem River and upper Manhattan in the distance, was the Hall of Fame of great Americans with their busts lined up in greeting for admiring visitors strolling through the semicircular colonnade and its extensions.

For many city dwellers who lacked the funds to send their children to live-in college campuses, this seemed a good alternative for so-called subway students such as myself. Two other considerations led me to the Heights: my father had graduated from the Heights in 1917 and wished me to follow in his footsteps, and my older brother had just been sent overseas by the U.S. Army, and my parents did not wish another absentee son at the same time.

So, it seemed, there was no logical choice for me to make other than attend the Heights. However, in terms of my using the Heights as a stepping stone to medical school, it was to prove a disaster. I soon learned that at least half of the matriculants in the University College of Arts and Science were premedical students and, given the demographics of New York City, the majority were Jewish. The biology department, in the person of its chairman, Horace W. Stunkard, took up the task of weeding out as many of them as possible so that at the end of four years, the number of Jewish premed students might be significantly reduced. A single D or F in any science would be enough to eliminate a student completely from any consideration for acceptance, given the degree of competition for medical school at the time.

Professor Stunkard was not an openly avowed anti-Semite, but it was not difficult to discern such an attitude by observing his behavior. His natural expression was a scowl, relieved only on those occasions when he waxed nostalgic about his happiest years, those in Berlin, where he studied in the thirties. One could not help wondering if this might have had something to do with the fact that it was at that time the Nazis were setting up shop and about to take over the country. I recently contacted another ex-Heightsman who had mentioned something about Stunkard in a book of his. The few sentences about this former professor were not unflattering, but later when I wrote the author, and we ended up corresponding, he mentioned another of our former professor's proclivities, the scheduling of examinations on Yom Kippur, the one day of the year when even the nonreligious Jew is likely to observe the holiday. Stunkard finally passed on at the age of 101, bringing to mind the adage about only the good dying young. As will be made clear, Stunkard was not alone in his discriminatory practices, but only a bizarre outcropping of the edifice of institutionalized anti-Semitism in the American medical educational establishment.

Actually, my own behavior in college did little to better my already slim chances of being accepted to medical school upon graduation. My father had something to do with this. He had a mid-nineteenth-century gentleman's view of the function of a college education. But his quaint Lord Chesterfieldian advice to his son was highly inappropriate for a modest dress salesman in the New York garment industry, with a son in a highly competitive situation and few other prospects for career success other than in one of the professions. I was advised by my father to become a "well-rounded person" in college, to participate fully in campus life and not become a drudge or bookworm, bogged down in schoolwork. Dutiful son that I was, I accepted this advice as gospel, and within the first two weeks of school had joined the campus newspaper, the glee club, the dramatic society and had pledged a fraternity.

Soon, in addition to attempting the adjustment to the academic demands of college after the relatively undemanding routine of high school, I was going to glee club rehearsals, stage managing a play, writing articles for the newspaper, and undergoing all kinds of time-consuming nonsense that pledging a fraternity entailed. Each night, thanks to all these activities, I arrived home well after ten to begin studying, hoping to recoup some additional study time on the upcoming weekend. Miraculously, I received no D's and failed no courses in college, not even Stunkard's biology course, but for the first three semesters came home will only B's and C's. Although the C's were replaced by A's in my later college career, the albatross of that initial mediocre showing still clung firmly about my neck. I emerged with a respectable but hardly impressive B average by the time I completed my senior year. This offered little hope of gaining me acceptance to medical school when other premeds in my class with B plus and A averages were being denied admission routinely and were going into dental school, law, accounting, or medical colleges in foreign countries where post-war American dollars were in high demand (Holland, Switzerland, and elsewhere).

My year of graduation, 1950, was a particularly difficult one for those intending to study medicine. The swelling of our student ranks by World War II veterans, taking advantage of the GI Bill to complete their education, was a major factor. Throughout the country they often constituted a high percentage of male student bodies. Everything else being equal, they would rightfully be granted first crack at medical school over those such as myself. The ratio of applicants to openings that year was one of the worst, if not *the* worst of modern times: approximately twenty-eight thousand applicants for seven thousand positions.

A one in four ratio for acceptance may not strike one as so terribly awful, considering the highly desirable nature of the positions in question (it has run from 1:2 to 1:3 in recent years), but it was not as simple as that.

The veteran factor has already been noted. Then there was the influence of geography. Most states tended, and still do, to favor their own residents. When the medical schools are state supported rather than private, this may even be mandated by law. But the number of medical schools, public and private, in any state can give a false impression about the ease of access to the aspiring premedical student. There may be only one medical school in a state, but if that state is sparsely populated, the applicant/acceptance ratio might be quite good. On the other hand, even though a state such as New York may have several private and public schools, and the total number of openings may seem large, the applicant pool is so much larger that the chances of acceptance are considerably less. In 1950, among the nearly three hundred graduates of the New York University Arts College, I estimated that at least half were undaunted premeds who had survived the screening process of the previous four years. Of these approximately 150 graduates, less than one in seven, would actually be admitted to an American medical school. I was not among them.

The reasons for the poor showing of the Heightsmen were not all related simply to the number of applicants and the number of slots available among New York's medical colleges. There was an overwhelming preponderance of Jews among our premedical contingent, and for a number of years, there had been a well-recognized and tolerated conspiracy to eliminate as many of "this kind" as possible from student and faculty positions in American medical education. Catholics, especially if they were of Italian background, also came in for their share of discrimination. Blacks were still too downtrodden to have access to medical schools (except for the black schools such as Howard and Meharry). Hispanics and women were not even considered as an afterthought for the most part. Not being Catholic, Italian, black, Hispanic, or female, I will confine my observations to the Jews.

In the early part of this century, especially in the Northeast, large numbers of Eastern European immigrants, many of them Jews, had settled in such cities as New York, Boston, and New Haven. As well documented in his book, *Joining the Club: A History of Jews and Yale*,[1] Dan Oren describes how college officials had become concerned about an increasing number of Jews infiltrating their student bodies. At Yale, for instance, in the undergraduate school, Jews constituted 5 percent of the enrollment in 1910, rising to 8 percent by 1921 with over 13 percent by 1925. Similar trends were becoming apparent at other upper-class bastions of higher education such as Princeton, Dartmouth, and Harvard. At Harvard in Boston between 1900 and 1922, the number of Jewish students had risen from 7 to 21 percent.

To counter this trend, the president of Harvard publicly proposed a quota system to limit this influx, but even in those less racially enlightened times, this kind of policy was considered a bit extreme, and following the adverse editorial attention the announcement engendered, the proposal was withdrawn— from public scrutiny. In the succeeding years, even through World War II and beyond, there was a tacit agreement among admissions officers of such institutions to keep a tight rein on the numbers of "undesirables" admitted. Certainly such restrictions had extended to 1950 as far as medical school admissions were concerned.

For privately funded colleges there were many dodges under which such discriminatory practices could be conducted. When "character and personality" in the choice of applicants wore a little thin, some schools claimed an obligation to cater to and then enroll the children of alumni, major contributors to endowment funds (and almost invariably WASPish). The desire for geographic diversity among the student body was another ploy. The significance that there were not a hell of a lot of Jewish cowboys in Montana and Wyoming was lost on no one, least of all the Jewish kids competing for the same college openings in their hometowns.

I recall many Jewish classmates, much brighter than I—Phi Beta Kappas, A averages and all that—who never had a chance in this country and went abroad to study or reluctantly gave up medicine altogether. Despite the odds, however, I still hoped to attend medical school. I mistakenly thought that my own contributions to campus life and friendly relationships with a number of faculty might compensate for my slow academic start, but they did not. One incident in particular brought this home to me.

I had appeared in a three character operetta with one pleasant chap a year ahead of me who was also premed. We actually toured the metropolitan area with our highly popular production over a two-year period. He had had the misfortune of either failing or getting a D (I forget exactly which) in that obstacle course, biology. Ordinarily a grade this low was a fatal blow to one's ambitions for medical school. But he had a charming Scottish name and a letter of recommendation from the professor who led the glee club to the head of the admissions committee at NYU-Bellevue, our sister college. He was accepted to the medical school. The following year I too had a letter, but no acceptance despite a much better academic record and a portfolio with many more activities, including the presidency of the honorary extracurricular society.

It was the same story everywhere. I recall an interview with Nobel Laureate Arthur Kornberg in which he told me that, among over two hundred bright students in his graduating class from the City College of New York, most of them Jewish, only five were accepted to medical school, he being among the few fortunate ones. At that time Columbia's College of Physicians and Surgeons had not accepted a single student from the City College of New York for ten years despite the Jacobi scholarship which provided full scholarship support for any graduate of that school attending Columbia's medical school.

Even after entering medical school, Kornberg met with similar discrimination. After winning honors for his performance as a first year student at Rochester, he was denied the opportunity for a research fellowship, one that would have been automatically granted to any non-Jew with such a record.

Jewish faculty often suffered similar discrimination when it came to appointments or promotions. Back at Yale, Louis Weinstein, a promising microbiologist, early in his career was told that he could not expect to rise beyond the rank of assistant professor in that department. Thanks to that policy he switched to medicine and became one of the outstanding infectious disease experts of our time.

It was bad enough to have the medical educational establishment against you, but when it included your own coreligionists, it was like pouring salt into a wound. The Jewish turncoat Milton Winternitz, a brilliant administrator and pathologist who served as dean at Yale's medical school between 1920 and 1935, was only the most bizarre example of this breed. At first he screened all applicants personally to weed out as many Jews as possible. Later, when the task became too burdensome for him, he appointed a committee on admissions with strict instructions to accept no more than five Jews and two Italian Catholics. Blacks were completely excluded from consideration as were women.

Stories about Winternitz's eccentricities and many outrages abound, but I am compelled to include here one example, whose source I am honor bound not to reveal. A Jewish student with superb academic credentials had appeared before Winternitz for an interview. The young man's somewhat swarthy complexion prompted the dean to say, "It's bad enough being a Jew, but being a Jew and looking like a nigger is even worse. Go elsewhere!" He did, and subsequently became a distinguished medical school professor.

Perhaps an even greater thorn in our collective Jewish student backsides was the house Hebrew of the American Medical Association, Dr. Morris Fishbein, whose prominent position made him a much greater factor on the medical scene than the loose cannon represented by someone like Winternitz. Secretary of the AMA, its public spokesman throughout the thirties and forties, and for many years the editor in chief of the *Journal of the American Medical Association*, the imperious Fishbein maintained a sublime indifference to the plight of his coreligionist students. There were a handful of other Jews who managed to attain positions of prominence in the medical establishment but, for the most part, were either too discouraged, fearful, or co-opted to attempt any reform.

Given the generally grim prospects confronting the vast majority of Jewish premedical students, they often grasped at any straw that might enhance their chances for admission. In my own fraternity there was one fellow a couple of years ahead of me who, I was told, had a wealthy physician uncle who had accumulated a valuable medical library. This was offered as a gift to one of the smaller medical colleges known for its chronic lack of funds and possibly venal inclinations. The gift was graciously accepted but not the nephew.

In my senior year, I had applied to about fifteen schools. As the rejections began to appear in the mailbox week after week, month after depressing month, I began to see the writing on the wall. But there was one hope. Parents such as mine were always looking for someone with influence who just might be willing to intervene on the part of their worthy son. Through charity work, my father had come into contact with a wealthy manufacturer who had been a great fund raiser for NYU-Bellevue. My father asked him for assistance. One evening some time later, I was brought by my father to some charity function to meet the great philanthropist. He placed his hand on my shoulder and smiled benignly.

"Allen, my boy, I am happy to tell you that next week you will be receiving a letter from NYU medical school."

I did; it was a rejection.

Why did people like me and my parents persist in following such a difficult pathway? The truth of the matter was that until recent years, there were few other opportunities open to bright, ambitious, young Jewish men. If their fathers had businesses, then the sons could be brought in. If the boys were inherently entrepreneurial, then they might find a way to start their own small businesses. Aside from this, only the professions—medicine, law, teaching—offered them a chance for future security and success. Executive training programs in large corporations, as we now know them, were few and far between and certainly not open to Jews and other ethnic minorities. Even for menial positions such as those in factories or in utilities such as the telephone company, Jews were excluded, especially when economic times were hard.

Some might consider my views on all this harsh and exaggerated. Dr. Leon Sokolof, a pathologist at the State University of New York at Stony Brook, has taken what might be considered a more balanced analysis of the Jewish quota system used in American medical schools earlier in this century. In a long and well-documented article that appeared in 1992, while he acknowledges that "old-fashioned anti-Semitism was one piece of the problem," he emphasizes economic factors and social attitudes as well.[2]

Professor Sokolof also notes the long historical connection of Jews to medicine and the rich tradition this represents. Nevertheless, the rising number of Jewish applicants to American medical schools in the earlier part of this century must surely have been a cause for alarm among admissions committees, largely gentile in composition. In 1934, for example, the secretary of the American Association of Medical Colleges reported that over 60 percent of the applications received were from Jewish students. Although this no doubt reflected the fact that Jewish applicants, conscious of the barriers against them, probably applied to a great many more schools than their gentile counterparts, the impression of an impending Yiddish Peril about to overwhelm them might have been understandable in the minds of medical school deans of the time. Nevertheless, the means employed to deal with this concern were hardly in line with the best American traditions of fair play and honesty.

Ironically, now that barriers against Jews have disappeared in many areas of American educational, business, and professional life, and Jewish physicians are well represented in many branches of medicine, especially in teaching and research, the percentage of Jewish youth entering medicine seems to have fallen. Only 8.6 percent of the first year entering class of 1988 actually identified themselves as Jewish.

Now, returning to my personal history: after the rejections in 1950, my year of graduation, my goal continued to be medical school. During my first post-college year, I attempted to obtain a research position at Columbia University's Presbyterian Hospital near my home in Washington Heights. I failed in this. The best I could come up with was a job running a messenger service at the posh Harkness Pavilion. Evenings I attended a chemistry class in quantitative analysis at City College in an attempt to bolster my academic standing. The result of my applications the second time around was the same.

At this point I had come to the conclusion that I simply was not ever going to become a doctor and that I might just as well accept the idea. With my flair for the theatrical, I turned to the entertainment world, which for the next two years pretty much amounted to backstage work for NBC television. Some creative outlet was found in off-Broadway acting and direction in my free time. In the spring of 1952, I was laid off at NBC and was about to take a job in summer stock when my ROTC (Reserve Officers' Training Corps) commission in the Air Force caught up with me. I was called up for two years of active duty at the height of the Korean War.

Early on in Transportation Officers School at Lowry Air Force Base in Colorado, where I was sent for training, a critical conversation turned my life around. At one of our bull sessions, a thirty-five-year-old reserve major who had also been called to active duty, informed the rest of us that he had always wanted to be a lawyer. Now, thanks to the Korean Veteran bill, which provided one and a half day's schooling support for every day of service, he would be able to attend law school following his tour of duty.

The thought that immediately came to my mind was "If that old man can go to law school at his age then when I get out, I can certainly try for medicine again." I was six months short of my twenty-third birthday at the time. Twenty-four months of service would translate into thirty-six months of support, the equivalent of four years of medical school. The monthly stipend would total $110 for all educational and living costs, hardly enough to meet all expenses, but with savings as an Air Force officer, working part time and perhaps on vacations during school years, with or without loans, I would be able to swing it, I thought.

What I was not sure of, at the time, was whether I still really wanted to become a physician, or whether I just wanted to prove to all those s.o.b.'s who had frustrated me that I could do the job.

During the second of my two years of active duty, I began the application process for the third time. Although I applied to about a dozen American schools, I had no real hope of being accepted by any of them. In fact, without illusions about my chances in the States, I had enrolled in the University of Amsterdam and was preparing to study Dutch when the acceptance arrived from the State University of New York—College of Medicine at New York, commonly known as Downstate in Brooklyn.

My interviewer had been Professor Chandler McCuskey Brooks, then head of the combined pharmacology and physiology departments at the old Henry Street campus near Borough Hall in downtown Brooklyn. I will never know what it was that impressed my benefactor: my determination or my all-American appearance in my powder blue Air Force uniform with the Eisenhower jacket. Maybe things had just loosened up enough in the admissions process to let me get through. In any event, I will always be grateful for the chance he offered me and am glad I had the opportunity of writing to him of this before his accidental death a few years back.

Following medical school came internship and residencies in San Francisco, a fellowship in cardiology in Utah, and a fairly successful academic career in New Jersey over the last three decades. I can thus tell this story with no taint of sour grapes to the flavor. The reason I am compelled to relate it is that in the 1990s our young people are so oblivious of this shameful record of American higher education. I mention past anti-Semitism to my students, and they look at me as if I were a creature from another planet, trying to communicate in some unintelligible tongue.

Their ignorance is understandable on two grounds. First, times have fortunately changed. Second, many of us who have experienced this aspect of American medicine have been so traumatized by it that it is too painful to recall. Dr. Kornberg originally withdrew his remarks on the subject after reviewing the initial draft of my interview for the book *Conversations in Medicine*[3] but relented after my appeal to his wife and sons helped convince him that it was a story that needed to be told. Other Jewish doctors I have interviewed were more adamant about concealing such past troubling experiences. One was Dr. Max(well) M. Wintrobe (1901–1986), for many years chairman of the Department of Medicine at the University of Utah School of Medicine and one of the world's premier hematologists.

As a rising star in medical research, Wintrobe was wooed away from Tulane to Johns Hopkins, the place where he had always dreamed of working as a young man. He and his wife arrived in Baltimore, and soon he was ushered into the dean's office where newly arriving faculty were given lists of available lodgings. The dean's secretary, after initially proffering the list to Wintrobe, had an afterthought. "Dr. Wintrobe, you're not Jewish by any chance?"

"I am."

"Oh, then this list is not for you," and it was withdrawn.

Although Wintrobe always recalled Hopkins as "a splendid place to work," he realized that he would never be offered the "top job" (chairmanship) there, that the best he could hope for was an associate professorship at some point in the far future. Socially, Baltimore was segregated along religious as well as racial lines, and the Wintrobes never had any social contacts with other, non-Jewish, faculty members during their stay. In 1943 they moved to Utah.

I believe that if current and future generations of Americans are made aware of such past experiences of some of the older ones among us, they might better understand our reaction to more recent developments. For example, past injustices to other groups, especially blacks, have been recognized, and some attempts have been made to correct them. My own school, the New

Jersey Medical School, has perhaps made the greatest strides toward this end when compared with other nonblack schools. Nonetheless, we are continually under attack for not doing enough.

All of which brings us to the case of the *Regents of the University of California* v. *Bakke*.

This case represents a signal episode in the affirmative action story and exhibits the many difficulties in interpretation and implementation that the program of affirmative action has entailed.

In the fall of 1972, Allan P. Bakke, a white male, then thirty-three years of age, applied for admission to the University of California Medical School at Davis. Despite his relatively advanced age for such an undertaking, his academic record and test scores were outstanding. He was denied admission to the freshman class that entered in the fall of 1973, and a second application for the following year was similarly rejected.

During this period there existed at Davis, as well as at a number of other medical schools throughout the country, a special admission program for disadvantaged minority students. Under the Davis program, there were sixteen of the one hundred places in the freshman class reserved for applicants meeting these particular specifications. Bakke did not qualify. Since many of the students admitted to the school under the program had academic records distinctly inferior to Bakke's, he claimed that his constitutional rights had been violated; that, in fact, by accepting students of a certain group with less adequate credentials than his own, the medical school at Davis was practicing reverse discrimination. He sued the University of California and won by a 6–1 decision when the case came before the California Supreme Court.

The University of California appealed the case to the United States Supreme Court, and it soon became an issue of national proportions. It was reported that in this case there were more friend of the court briefs filed with the Court by interested agencies than in any other case in its previous history. The Supreme Court, perhaps wisely, straddled the debate in its decision. It came down against fixed quotas being set, as had been the case at Davis, but supported other measures to promote affirmative action in the interests of disadvantaged minorities. Bakke was quietly admitted to medical school and graduated without incident.

It is more than of passing interest that Jewish organizations, so often allied with blacks in the past, aligned themselves in opposition to the National Association for the Advancement of Colored People and other black civil rights organizations on the Bakke case. (Bakke, incidentally, is not Jewish.) Undoubtedly, the setting up of any educational quota systems was anathema to Jews, given their own past experience. Amazingly, this was lost on many people who should have realized the ominous implications of such actions.

In our own student body, a young woman activist approached me at one point. Since women constituted over half our population, she insisted, they deserved to have similar proportionate representation in medicine as well as other professions. To me this sounded like quotas all over again. She seemed surprised on learning the logical extension of her argument: since Jews constituted only 3 percent of the population and since she was Jewish as well as female, her category entitled her kind to only 1.5 percent of medical school admissions. In her class of approximately one hundred students, there were already three Jewish women. I suggested that if she really believed in what she was saying, then the only moral thing to do was to resign her own place in the class to restore a just balance. Absurd? Of course, but very revealing to what excesses such reverse discriminatory practices could lead. In more recent times I see prejudice rearing its ugly head once again as some of the remarks that used to be routinely directed at "pushy Jews" are now applied to hard working and eminently deserving Americans of Asian background who are now beginning to come to the fore in competition for prized positions in higher education.

In my own lifetime I have had the opportunity to view the issue from both sides of the fence. I have already written of my experiences as a medical school applicant; I now turn to my experiences as a faculty member and medical school admissions officer.

In the academic year of 1970–71 I was chosen to be a member of the admissions committee of the New Jersey Medical School. The following year I was asked by the dean to serve as chairman of the committee, and I accepted. It was an ironic turn of events if there ever was one, although one of my psychiatrist friends to whom I confided this impression assured me that it was "inevitable."

The early seventies marked a turning point in medical school admissions policies. The successes of the Civil Rights movement of the sixties had awakened medical school administrations and faculties to the past injustices suffered by blacks, Hispanics, and other disadvantaged minorities. At our own school, now located in the middle of the black section of Newark, the near absence of black faces among our student body and faculty was an extreme embarrassment. We quickly moved to the forefront in instituting programs to correct such inequities. In retrospect we made mistakes, as well meaning as they were, and these mistakes, as well as the responses to them, point up the misconceptions that were and still are so prevalent about the Bakke case and similar issues.

In 1969 and 1970, for many medical schools attempting to begin such special admissions programs, the problem was finding sufficient numbers of disadvantaged minority students (in our case, mainly blacks) qualified to begin the study of medicine. Until that time most blacks attending college tended to seek careers in teaching, social work, and the arts. The professions such as medicine were, with good reason, often assumed to be inaccessible to these young people. When the doors of the medical schools were suddenly swung open, there was a dearth of adequately prepared candidates to choose from among these students. While the Ivy League schools, with awe-inspiring reputations and equally awe-inspiring financial support programs, skimmed off the academic cream, other institutions, such as ours, were left to evaluate what remained.

What happened in Newark was a painful experiment, which in our naïveté at the time we had hardly envisioned. Because of the desire to meet our moral obligation, we decided to accept some of those remaining in the minority pool who were on shaky academic ground but who we felt had at least some reasonable chance of meeting the challenge of the medical school curriculum. Approximately a dozen entered in the fall of 1971, just as I assumed chairmanship of the committee. Many proved within the first year to have considerable difficulty with their work. In the spring of 1972 some were required by the promotions committee to repeat the year. Several were advised that they would be dropped from the rolls of the school. Although we regretted this action, we realized that we had put some of these students in an impossible position, but at least a beginning had been made as we rejoiced in the success of the others.

When news of the dismissals reached the black community in Newark, a near riot ensued. They looked upon our initial acceptance of the black students as only a cruel deception. They believed that we never had intended to pass them on to the second year from the day we had offered them places in the first. Pressure mounted on the administration of the school to reverse these decisions. At one point the faculty council was physically imprisoned in its meeting room for several hours as black students and community activists manned the doors. Although the reaction of the community was understandable, the subsequent reversal of the council's actions had a severe demoralizing effect upon faculty who rightly viewed their decision-making powers as having been taken from them. Many basic science faculty, upon whom the heaviest burden fell as instructors for the first two years of medical school and who did not have the option of just going into the private practice of medicine if they lost their jobs, simply decided to pass all these students through and let someone else deal with the problem later.

This provided a long fuse for another bomb, one that exploded in the spring of 1976 when the first two senior students in the history of the school, both black, were not allowed to graduate with their class because of academic difficulties. Passage of the National Board examination, requisite to state licensure, was a hurdle that some of these students were never to overcome.

It should be emphasized that the number of students involved were relatively few. An increasing number of the disadvantaged minority pool have proved to be fully up to the curriculum. For those of this group hoping to embark upon medical careers while still in undergraduate school, a Students for Medicine program at our school has provided preliminary preparation and evaluation to avoid the disastrous misjudgments of the past.

One might ask if specific affirmative action goals/quotas are necessary if improved representation of these groups is to persist? About twenty years ago when such programs were first being instituted, I was made uneasy by the obvious (to me) quotas they included. Nevertheless, I convinced myself that some activism toward these goals was necessary for the time being but that some day they might no longer be needed in a forward moving and enlightened society. In 1992, however, figures provided by the American Medical Association indicate that representation is still less than it should be. Meanwhile many whites contend that "It's better than it was," while most blacks insist "It's no where near where it should be."

The debate goes on, and California once again provides a venue for the conflicting interests involved in access to not only the study of medicine, but all forms of higher education. On July 20, 1995, the University of California Board of Regents voted to end a thirty-year policy of utilizing affirmative action goals in decisions affecting student admissions. Obviously spurred by increasing white resentment about the perceived preferential treatment of blacks and Hispanics and led by an opportunistic and politically ambitious governor, the regents sought by this action to preserve for the future whatever they could of white higher educational turfdom within the state. But while they preached in favor of strictly academic criteria and individual accomplishment, they obviously overlooked the growing dominance of Asian-Americans among them in higher education. As of 1995, 40 percent or more of the students at U.C. in Berkeley were of Asian-American extraction. Ironically, the new color blind criteria for admission to the University of California campuses, obviously devised to benefit white applicants vis-à-vis blacks and Hispanics, will probably work to further exclusion of whites from these highly desirable seats of higher education as Asian-American students with superior academic credentials complete the process of crowding them out even more effectively than the favoring of disadvantaged minorities ever did.

Even on the eastern seaboard, in Boston, hardly a major settlement of Asiatic immigrants, the trend is unmistakable. At the Massachusetts Institute of Technology, the director of admissions wrote me that in 1995 28 percent of the 1130 freshmen admitted were of Asian-American background. These 322 Asian-American students represented almost twice the number of African-Americans, Native Americans, Mexican-Americans, Puerto Rican-Americans and other Hispanic-Americans *combined*.

I, for one, do not believe that Asians are basically more intelligent than Westerners. The Japanese attained their economic hegemony in large part by capitalizing on technical developments they imported from the United States and Europe. I do believe that our students of Asian background are often harder working and more strongly motivated than their white counterparts—just like the Jewish students of fifty years ago. If they are succeeding so well by dint of these admirable qualities, we should rejoice that they are American citizens and will contribute to advancing the social and economic future for all of us. I also believe, with some sadness and trepidation, that I may be among a minority of whites that so firmly hold this view.

As I look back upon the road I personally followed toward the study and practice of medicine, I am conscious of the fact that the very collegiate exploits that doomed my scholastic performance as an undergraduate ended up enhancing my performance as a pedagogue. As a frequent lecturer, I attribute my public-speaking skill to the ability to project my voice effectively, a gift acquired from those days of performing in the glee club and chapel choir. This quality was reinforced by those nights on stage with the Hall of Fame Players, and from that training ground I also learned to bring some theater into my current tasks, making lectures and conferences entertaining as well as informative. Also, knocking off all those stories at the *Heights Daily News* speeded my typing considerably, and who knows, the who-what-when-where-why inculcated in the Heights newsroom may have enabled me to get this long story—and others—just a little straighter than might otherwise have been the case.

Notes

1. Oren DA. *Joining the Club: A History of Jews and Yale.* New Haven: Yale Univ. Press, 1986.
2. Sokolof L. The rise and decline of the Jewish quota in medical school admissions Bull. NY Acad Med 1992; 68:497–518.
3. Weisse AB. *Conversations in Medicine: The Story of Twentieth-Century American Medicine in the Words of Those Who Created It.* New York: New York Univ. Press, 1984.

2

Betrayal

IN MEDICINE, as in other scientific disciplines, the roles of mentor and student have been critical in the development of a body of knowledge as well as in the development of cadres of experts who have contributed to the well being and advancement of society. Earlier in our national history, however, throughout the nineteenth and early twentieth centuries, when North American medicine was still emerging from its backwater status, those American physicians with the will and wherewithal to advance their own knowledge often had to travel abroad to acquaint themselves with the latest developments in medical research and practice.

Europe was invariably their destination, with Germany, especially, the source of innovation and expertise. Not only practicing physicians ventured abroad; there were also those we now call basic scientists—physiologists, biochemists, microbiologists—who sought out centers of learning in order to equip themselves to elevate standards of teaching and research back home. In Leipzig, for example, the kindly, avuncular Karl Ludwig (1816–1895) trained over two hundred advanced pupils in physiology over the course of his long career. Many of these were Americans who returned to the States to head departments of physiology in major medical schools throughout the country. They, in turn, spawned their own progeny of teachers and researchers in the field.

There have also been famous "loners" in science, individuals with neither the taste nor talent for incubating the careers of their juniors. Isaac Newton, perhaps, might represent the quintessential example of such a one. More recently, Alexis Carrel, the Franco-American who contributed so much to the development of cardiovascular surgical techniques early in this century and was awarded a Nobel prize in recognition of this, might be considered another.

However, the careers of many more medical scientists might better fit the description of researcher-teacher, and it is to them we are most indebted for the growth and quality of medicine over the last century or more.

As a cardiologist, I have been particularly interested in circulatory physiology, and one of my heroes in the field has always been Carl J. Wiggers (1883–1963) who headed the Department of Physiology at Case Western Reserve from 1918 until 1953. From his laboratory emerged many of the major figures in circulatory physiology of this century. In clinical cardiology, similar lineages were established as exemplified by the trainees of such pioneers as Paul Dudley White in Boston and the Johns Hopkins pediatric cardiologist, Helen B. Taussig.

Parallels abound in many other fields of medicine. A hematologist might be described as having come out of the laboratory of the great Max Wintrobe at the University of Utah or that of William Damoshek in Boston. Many other examples might easily be cited.

The most distinctive lineages, perhaps, are those that have been established by the great surgeons of the century. Johns Hopkins, by most estimates, was the leading American medical school at the beginning of the century. There William S. Halsted headed the surgical department and under his guidance a number of surgical subspecialties were born; not least was neurosurgery, fathered by Harvey W. Cushing. In later years at the same institution, Dr. Alfred Blalock, deviser with Helen Taussig of the famous "blue baby operation" that saved or prolonged the lives of so many children with cyanotic congenital heart disease, trained generations of surgeons who established their own dynasties at medical schools throughout the land. Owen H. Wangensteen was elevated to the surgical chair at the University of Minnesota at the tender age of thirty-one in 1930. During his thirty-seven-year tenure in that post, he spawned over a hundred future professors of surgery, many of whom came to head their own departments at other prominent medical institutions.

Note the terms I have used to describe the master/pupil relationship and the results of such collaborations: "gave birth to," "spawned," "lineage," "fathered," and "dynasty." Up and coming figures might also have been described as "one of so-and-so's boys" or a "so-and-so man." Given the exclusion of women from positions of medical authority during this time, it was almost always a man-to-man relationship and the terms describing it most suggestive of a kind of bloodline from one medical generation to the next. Indeed, in the best of circumstances, these were and still are parent-child affairs, and the young men and women entering into them yield not only many years of their lives but their autonomy and trust to those who will be responsible for molding their professional lives in the years to come.

We often read or hear of such relationships described in glowing terms. Seldom documented are the instances where those in positions of power and prestige have abused and sometimes even professionally crippled the young people who had entrusted themselves to such flawed or aberrant masters. The best known stories concerning such misbehavior have centered on the best known reward for scientific excellence, the Nobel Prize in Physiology or Medicine. The best known of these involves the discovery of insulin.

In 1921, while working in the Department of Physiology at the University of Toronto, Frederick Banting, a young surgeon, and his student-assistant, Charles H. Best, were the first to isolate insulin for the treatment of diabetes. However, in 1923, when the Nobel Committee named the recipients of the prize for that year, it was John R. McLeod, the head of the department, who was chosen to share the award with Banting rather than Best. Banting felt that McLeod had unjustly deprived Best of his rightful reward and showed his disapproval by making public his sharing of the monetary prize with Best and refusing to attend the award ceremonies in Stockholm.

As an example of betrayal, this, of course, is an imperfect one. Although McLeod might have been held accountable for the mistreatment of Best, the true mentor in this case was Banting who so admirably came to the defense of his young protégé.

Another notable case involved the discovery of streptomycin, the first effective antibiotic for the treatment of tuberculosis and a major milestone in the history of infectious diseases. It was Selman Waksman, a soil biologist at Rutgers University, who received a Nobel Award for this in 1952. The actual bench work that led to the discovery, however, was performed by a graduate student, Albert Schatz, at no little risk to himself dealing with potentially lethal organisms long hours under rather primitive conditions by today's standards. Schatz brought suit against Rutgers, but was unsuccessful, and for years in many quarters was merely thought an ungrateful malcontent. Recently, however, his contributions have finally received their just recognition.

Such stories punctuate many aspects of medical discovery and, when they involve achievements of such magnitude as insulin and streptomycin, naturally draw considerable public attention. Fortunately, at times the end result of such abuses may not be negative. Charles Best, for example, went on to a very successful career in physiology and ended his life as one of the great figures in the field. Schatz, despite many years of suffering the injustice dealt him by the system, finally received the recognition due him.

Less well recognized than these major stories of medical history are the many instances of master-pupil discord that have occurred in less heroic settings. Yet, the despair felt by these acolytes, who have suffered at the hands of their professional fathers, is just as valid; the cutting off or extinguishing of a medical research career, even when earth-shaking discoveries are not involved, is just as devastating to those at the receiving end. This is one such story.

It begins at a time when I considered myself very fortunate in having obtained a fellowship position with an outstanding cardiologist at the University of Utah School of Medicine. He was well versed in the clinical as well as the research aspects of this burgeoning discipline. Recently out of a residency in internal medicine, I was eager to become involved in some aspects of cardiovascular research. This, after all, was during the sixties when the post-Sputnik flowering of American medical research was in its fullest bloom.

"Publish or perish" was already on the minds of all who envisioned pursuing such a career, and another trainee and I were anxious to get something into print and achieve that first rung on the academic ladder. We had come across a patient with an interesting problem at Salt Lake General Hospital where we worked and were in the process of writing it up as a case report, fully intending to present it to our professor for his comments and suggestions before submitting it for publication. Before we had completed the first draft, he accosted us one day on the hospital grounds simply fuming with indignation. Who in hell did we think we were, going behind his back to do such a thing? Several expletives later, we knew that the slightest initiative on our parts would never again be tolerated. Needless to add, we proceeded no further.

As a professor myself today, I would simply be delighted if two of my fellows surprised me with such initiative, independent of my prodding. I would be inclined to embrace them with gratitude and admiration since, too often, I find that those presently in subspecialty training seem more intent on seeking good leads for practice opportunities rather than ways to expand our medical knowledge. I was not to have the option of proceeding freely on my own during the course of my own remaining months of specialty training.

My next attempt at independent research involved a young pregnant woman with no prior history of cardiac disease who was found to have a potentially serious irregularity of the heartbeat, ventricular tachycardia. When the arrhythmia was detected during a routine prenatal checkup, I was assigned to treat her and follow her throughout the remainder of the pregnancy and delivery. I began to review the literature on such a rare occurrence—ventricular tachycardia during pregnancy in an otherwise normal individual—and was able to find only two previous reports. Samuel Bellet, a prominent Philadelphia cardiologist of the time, had reported one case in 1931, and the only previous documentation of a case had come from the father of cardiology himself, Sir James Mackenzie, in Great Britain ten years earlier. Surely my own case merited inclusion in the medical literature, I thought.

I closely followed the woman through her successful labor and delivery and then during a four-month period following this when she had no further evidence of a disordered heart rhythm despite the withdrawing of medication. I took pains to conceal all this from my chief before approaching him with the tentative suggestion that I write up the case with him.

"I don't care very much for case reports," he growled. "They clutter up the literature." But he gave me the go-ahead—temporarily.

The draft I presented with him as coauthor, even though he had had nothing to do with the case, the research, or the write-up, was returned to me with a number of comments, none of them flattering and some outrightly insulting. Still, corrections could be made, and they were. What I thought might be the final draft was submitted some weeks later. It was returned with a final comment: If we were really to be sure that the woman's arrhythmia was related to the pregnancy, then we should observe her for a recurrence during her next pregnancy before assuming it to be a matter of cause and effect. I noted to myself that such a requirement had been no impediment to the two previous reports, but then the previous authors had a lot more autonomy than I did at the time.

The obstacle that had been placed in my own path was insurmountable. I had less than a year to go in my training program, and I would soon be leaving the area. In any event, the lady in question had not the slightest intention of becoming pregnant again, not even in the interests of medical science and my own career. Dead end.

The next few months offered a reprieve for me and the other fellows in cardiology. Our chief had taken a sabbatical leave in Europe and would be out of our hair and off our backs for long enough for us to get on with any other projects we had in mind.

It was during this time that I became interested in certain aspects of normal heart sounds and certain misconceptions about them that I found were prevalent among the medical community. I began to record these sounds in normal subjects and sort out the relationship of the intensity of some components to others. This was certainly not in a league with the discovery of insulin or streptomycin but was one of the myriad of relatively minor matters that, when added up, contribute to the accuracy and entirety of our medical knowledge.

By the time my chief had returned to Salt Lake, I had accumulated seventy-five such studies to show him. It was not enough, he opined. I was then in my last month of fellowship and on my way back East to become an instructor at the Seton Hall School of Medicine (now the New Jersey Medical School). As soon as I arrived at my new post, I began to collect additional subjects and send revised manuscripts to my former chief.

I soon had 100 cases; not enough. Then I had 125; still not enough to satisfy him. Then 140; again a turndown at my former place of training. At this point, I balked. I wrote back with a final draft indicating that I was not prepared to spend the rest of my professional life collecting additional cases for this single project. If the paper, in its final form, did not match up to his standards, I would not presume to embarrass him by including him as an author. His reply indicated that this certainly was not the case and that I should proceed with submission of the paper for publication.

By this time I was well into my first year at my new job, and I had been fortunate enough to obtain additional professional input into the project. An older cardiologist at Seton Hall had come on board and offered helpful suggestions, an engineer at Bell Telephone had rigged up a little device for me to get more precise recordings of sound intensity, and a statistical whiz at my new institution had offered to help out in this aspect of analysis. Certainly they deserved their share in the authorship.

I submitted the manuscript to a prominent cardiology journal where my ex-chief just happened to sit on the editorial board. To this day I am not sure what it was that I did to incur his wrath once again, but I suspect it was something as minor as listing him among the authors in a position not to his liking. Be that as it may, within a few weeks of the paper's submission, I received a scathing letter damning my impertinence at having placed his name on a paper in which he had played no part in the conception or execution at any time. He demanded immediate removal of his name from the manuscript. Completely dumbfounded by the viciousness of these uncalled for remarks, I had no choice but to write a follow-up letter to the editor in chief of the journal, explaining that, as a result of some misunderstanding, my former chief did not feel it appropriate that he be listed as a coauthor.

If you were that editor in chief, what would your response be to such a letter? Obviously smelling a nonexistent rat, he rejected the paper. When the manuscript was returned with the covering rejection letter, I sort of expected it, but what I did not envision was that it would provoke so many tears of anger and frustration at having been so unfairly and cruelly treated by a mentor to whom I had so completely entrusted myself and depended upon for support.

The paper, minus one of the original authors, was submitted to another reputable journal, accepted without need for revision, and I am pleased to add, is still occasionally cited in the literature more than twenty years after its publication. Since that time I have published many other research papers, commentaries, and several books, so my story has not really ended as a sad one. On the other hand, for much of the last thirty years or so, what modest research I have accomplished has in no small part been to demonstrate to the s.o.b. of my youth (and to *myself*) that I was really worth my salt.

The depressing part of the story is that this twisted misanthrope occupied a preeminent position in the field for many decades. How many other budding investigators, less determined than I but perhaps much more gifted, were crushed in the process? There are a few, like myself, who were fortunate enough to survive the experience, and conversations with them parallel my own memories of that period. But the record of that laboratory documents the burden of its guiding spirit in that so few of those who trained under him ever chose to remain within the academic community, compared to similar laboratories elsewhere in the United States.

It is possible to outlive such hurtful early experiences. It is also possible for some who have undergone them to take the philosophical approach, to forgive even when they cannot forget. I was told the story of an old friend from another laboratory, a laboratory even more distinguished than the one in which I had trained. It was headed by a man internationally recognized for his integrity and kindness as well as his ability. (His father had been a minister!) It was the same man with whom my friend left a coauthored manuscript for final touches when he departed for a new position elsewhere. The next time my friend saw this paper, was when it appeared in a journal of great repute—now under one name, that of his former chief. It was my friend, of course, who had been responsible for almost all the work and writing of the paper before he left. Incredibly, he bears no animus toward the man who deceived him and even does him honor.

As for my own experience, I take comfort in having survived it. But forget? Forgive? Never.

3

The Vanishing Male

THERE IT WAS in black and white: another nail in the coffin of our once vaunted masculinity. My recent issue of *Science* featured a report demonstrating that in the breeding of a certain kind of wasp there were bacteria that killed off only the male eggs of the species.

The deadly courting behavior of the black widow spider is common knowledge, of course, and I recently learned that the praying mantis female also disposes of her mate in the act of procreation. I have no doubt that, if we search long and hard enough, we will find literally thousands of species of insects in which, if not outrightly killed in the act of creation, the males are, at the very least, severely ostracized thereafter—much like the drones in the beehive after they have served their purpose.

As one ascends the evolutionary ladder, things don't improve very much for the males of the species. Among birds, although there are instances of lifelong pairing, more often than not, during mating season the male simply "struts and frets his hour upon the stage and then is heard no more." A nature film addict, I recall the contortions of a perfectly splendid bird of paradise who did everything but the ornithological equivalent of standing on his head (he hung upside down from a branch) in a futile attempt to attract a potential mate. After she had waltzed off with a rival, there he was in his magnificent plumage "all dressed up with no place to go."

The rutting of elk and the competition of rams seem to be favorites of the television nature photographer, and there are endless encounters of mature male elk wrestling with their horns locked in deadly embrace and rams whose ear-shattering head bashings set the very walls of my living room reverberating. Some of these males will wind up with harems, but my sympathy invariably goes to the losers who must wind up with what can only be described as a terrible headache with nary an aspirin in sight for relief.

A popular arctic sequence featured the mating of polar bears, among the largest and most majestic carnivores on earth. Soon after being impregnated, the female tunnels into the ground for a winter of gestation, finally emerging in the spring with two or three adorable little snow-white cubs to keep her company. Meanwhile, Papa Bear has been banished to wander alone in the dark and frigid icy wasteland.

In Joy Adamson's book, *Born Free*, I was impressed that it was the lioness that took the initiative in the mating game and not the so-called King of the Beasts who, like the polar bear, was, at least for some time after the birth of the cubs, excluded from the family hearth.

My fascination with mating habits extends to humans, where, strangely enough, we seem to actively contradict the practices so common to other mammals. I have heard of a primitive tribe in which, when the mother goes into labor, the father mimics all the responses of the painful process, screaming and writhing on the ground, while the mother, hidden off somewhere in the bush, quietly "delivers the goods." But even modern man, with the approval and sometimes instigation of his spouse, comes awfully close to this. With jointly practiced birth exercises during the pregnancy and his active participation as a one-man cheering squad during delivery, he is getting closer and closer to the act. Bringing up baby is also becoming a joint effort, and, with the increasing trend of two wage earners in the home, this is all to the good. But how about the rest of the human male condition?

The biological fragility of man, when compared to woman, is a fact of life. We are more subject to accidental death, early onset coronary disease, and other life-threatening catastrophes. The life expectancy tables of the insurance companies leave no doubt about it, and the hordes of excess widows over widowers attest to it. Nature, as if to attempt some sort of compensation for this preordained attrition, allows for a slight surplus of males over females among human births, but it doesn't seem to make much difference fifty years or so down the line.

Since men and women share a common society, the temptation to compare their accomplishments, whatever their life span, is irresistible. As a physician, educator, and writer, I tend to emphasize the intellectual aspects of human achievement. I am forced to conclude that, in many instances, the women win hands down. I graduated from high school as the second highest ranking boy—but there were a half-dozen girls whose academic records outshone both that of the valedictorian (in those days always the highest ranking boy student) and myself. As I have observed my students in medical school and the medical house staff under my supervision, I see the women with greater representation than the men among the best and brightest.

As I glance briefly into other fields of endeavor, I see women as equal to men in literature. Music, art, and business have been almost exclusively male preserves historically, but how much of this is due to nature and how much to nurture? In youth there are a few fleeting years when we are very conscious of the fact that males can run faster, jump higher, and lift heavier weights, but, over the span of an entire lifetime, this diminishes in importance.

How do other contemporary men feel about it? The "About Men" feature that used to appear from time to time in the Sunday magazine section of the *New York Times* provided an interesting but often troubling reflection of masculine attitudes. So few of the stories were triumphant, and I don't recall a single one that was really outrightly funny. There were a scattering of fond father-son memories and recollections of evanescent exploits on playing fields, in gymnasia, or somewhere outdoors. On the whole, though, they seemed to speak mainly of loneliness, of lost opportunities, lost ambition, lost loves, and lost illusions.

Personally, I consider myself fortunate but cannot really explain why. To twist a phrase from the Rodgers and Hammerstein ditty in *Flower Drum Song*, I have just enjoyed being a man.

I recall a conversation I had over thirty years ago with a Cajun from Louisiana, a young Air Force officer who had been called to active duty with me during the Korean conflict. We were billeted together for a time. He was a real charmer, and his exploits with the ladies were the envy of us all. Nevertheless, he was gnawed by doubts that he had yet to find himself in his chosen profession of engineering. As he expressed these doubts to me that night, he also told me that he comforted himself with another thought: that at the moment of his conception, it was he who was the sperm that had won out over the many thousands of others vying for admission to that one available egg.

"Just think," he mused, "I beat out all those other guys! So I must be really special after all."

Perhaps he had something there.

4

Pneumocystis and Me

The Small Joys and Great Satisfactions of Medical Sleuthing

Before I am finished, you may have learned more about *Pneumocystis* pneumonia and the bug that causes it (*Pneumocystis carinii*) than you ever needed or wanted to know. So be forewarned but not, I hope, forearmed because I trust that by the time I have finished, you will find what I have had to say as fascinating and as much fun as it was for me in the process of digging it out.

One day not long ago, upon completing general ward rounds as part of my duties as an attending physician, I realized that I must have supervised the care of over a hundred patients with Pneumocystis carinii pneumonia. It also suddenly dawned upon me that here I was, treating the most common opportunistic infection in AIDS and probably the most frequent cause of death from the disease, and I wasn't really sure about the name of the parasite (now thought to be a fungus) that caused it.

"Where does the name 'Pneumocystis carinii' come from?" I wondered aloud to my house staff.

The first part was easy. We all figured out that "Pneumocystis" referred to cysts in the lung. What we could not be sure about, however, was the derivation of "carinii." When I approached our infectious disease people and pulmonary specialists, there were similar doubts. The most likely source of the term, in the minds of those queried, was the anatomical carina, the point at which the trachea branches off into the main right and left bronchi of the lungs. Perhaps the pneumonia witnessed on X Ray by earlier investigators often seemed to be located predominantly in areas of the lung that were centrally located in this pattern.

I was not convinced, and before I knew it, I was plunged into the chaotic world of parasitic taxonomy. The Swede Carl von Linné (1707–1778), Linnaeus to you and me, began the process of Latinizing the names of plants and animals in a systematic way. It is generally agreed that he did quite well in botany but that his efforts in zoology left much to be desired. In parasitology, especially, there seems to be no rhyme or reason.

In naming these creatures, one could use the anatomic site infected (*Fasciola hepatica, Trichomonas vaginalis, Ancylostoma duodenale, Enterobius vermicularis*); the susceptible host (*Tococara canus, Trypanosoma equinum*); or even the geographic location where the parasite is found (*Ancylostoma braziliense, Trypanosoma gambiense, Trypanosoma rhodesiense, Schistosoma japonicum*).

The shape of the organism has been used on occasion: *Trichinella spiralis, Diphyllobothrium latum* for example. The names of scientists can be used for taxonomic purposes as demonstrated by the presence of Manson, Wucherer, and Bancroft in *Schistosoma mansoni* and *Wuchereria bancrofti*.

Trypanosoma cruzi has a special significance in the present discussion. The word "cruzi" might suggest some anatomical aspect of the parasite at first glance, but it actually refers to Oswaldo Cruz, for whom Carlos Chagas named the disease, honoring the chief of his department who had sent him into the Brazilian jungle to investigate a certain type of affliction that had descended upon the railway workers there as well as the local inhabitants. Chagas was to prove a major figure in my growing obsession with Pneumocystis carinii.

My first clue that the second part of the name did not refer to any anatomical structure came from an exhaustive review of Pneumocystis carinii pneumonia in 1957 by future Nobelist D. Carleton Gajdusek,[1] and to which I had been referred by one of our microbiologists. There it was, number 162 among the 204 references: Carini, A. Formas de eschizogonia do Trypanosoma Lewisi—in the Archives of the Society of Medicine and Surgery of São Paulo published in 1910. Carini was a man, and now I determined to find out all about him.

The first thing to do was to locate the original article, and a request for this was made through the Inter-Library Loan office at our medical school library. I also wanted some biographical data on Carini. For this I went to the membership directory of the Federation of American Societies for Experimental Biology. Basic scientists residing in foreign countries are occasionally members of one of the groups of biological scientists making up the federation. Could there be a likely candidate in Brazil?

Indeed there was. A lady Ph.D. was currently working at the Oswaldo Cruz Institute in Rio de Janeiro. I wrote and faxed her simultaneously. I also wrote to the laboratory in São Paulo where Carini had worked for many years.

As I awaited responses to these initial queries, I pondered about other potential sources of information. The name of Ben Kean popped into my mind. He had given a very informative and entertaining grand rounds for us years before and might still be at Cornell's Department of Tropical Medicine even though I imagined he must be close to eighty by this time if not older. A phone call across the river from New Jersey was easy enough to make.

Within moments of his answering the phone, I knew I had hit the mother lode.

"Carini? Oh yes, Antonio Carini was an Italian who worked in Brazil for about thirty-five years before he returned home. I'll mail you some stuff about him." I then heard him gruffly shouting to his secretary to pull out this and that to send to Dr. Weisse in Newark. Now deceased, Dr. Kean turned out to be to tropical medicine what I. F. Stone was to political reporting and Bill Mazer is to the world of sports: a walking encyclopedia.

Much of what I came to learn about Carini and Pneumocystis ultimately came from Kean or from leads provided by him. The reprints he sent me were chock full of important information about Pneumocystis and its discovery. I was also referred to Dr. Kean's wonderful book of reminiscences that I was still waiting to get to read.[2] Sure enough, Carini and Chagas are in it. So here's the story:

In 1909 Carlos Chagas (1879–1934) emerged from several years in the Brazilian jungle and published the results of his research which demonstrated for the first time that there was an American form of African sleeping sickness (although chronically the heart is more often affected than the nervous system and occasionally the gut).[3] We now call it Chagas' Disease although Chagas named it Trypanosoma cruzi in honor of his chief in Rio, Oswaldo Cruz, whom he would succeed as director of the Oswaldo Cruz Institute following the other's untimely death at the age of forty-five in 1917.

Now, in drawing the various forms exhibited during the life cycle of the parasite as observed under the microscope after he had obtained them from the lungs of infected guinea pigs, Chagas mistakenly included some rounded forms that were not *T. cruzi*, but actually forms of a coexistent infection, one that would later come to be known as Pneumocystis carinii.

A year later, in 1910, there appeared that report of Antonio Carini (1872–

1950) who was studying another flagellate, *Trypanosoma lewisi*, in rats. It appears that he made the same mistake that Chagas did in identifying some cystic structures as part of the life cycle of *T. lewisi* rather than as a separate pathogen.

In 1912, two French investigators, the Delanoës, also working with T. lewisi in rats, demonstrated that the "cysts of Carini" represented a new, previously unrecognized parasite.[4] In deference to the Italian-Brazilian's early description, they named it Pneumocystis carinii.

Why not *Pneumocystis chagasi*? Probably because Chagas' report concerned guinea pigs also infected with T. cruzi while the Delanoës made their observations in rats concurrently infected with T. lewisi as did Carini.

Although originally described as a parasitic invader of other mammals, Pneumocystis gradually established itself in humans as well. The first human cases were reported in 1942 as atypical interstitial pneumonias with additional reports, mainly in premature infants, as summarized by Gajdusek. Immunosuppression as a result of cancer chemotherapy and organ transplantation enabled Pneumocystis to gain a firmer foothold among us. Finally, with the advent of AIDS, it has become an almost constant companion to the retrovirus that assumed epidemic proportions throughout the world.

Although his name is attached to the disease that, in terms of the current medical literature, undoubtedly overshadows everything else he ever published, Carini was strangely overlooked in the only major account of Brazilian medical history that I was able to locate. In a book by Renato C. Bacellar on Brazil's contributions to tropical medicine,[5] Adolfo Lutz (1885–1940), Oswaldo Cruz, and Carlos Chagas are represented as the three great figures of this tradition. Perhaps so: they all played important roles in setting up the facilities for the investigation and control of such diseases among Brazil's inhabitants. However, among the dozens of lesser figures listed in the book's appendix, Carini's name does not even appear. I don't believe it was because Carini was not a native Brazilian; Lutz's birthplace was Rio, true, but both his parents were Swiss, and he spent all of his formative years in Europe. Yet, in spite of over thirty-five years honorable service at the Pasteur Institute in São Paulo, which he headed as director for a number of these years, inexplicably Carini's only mention in the book is in a passing reference to a paper he published with another man, not on the disease for which his name is now recalled, knowingly or not, but for his identification of the Bauru ulcer in Oriental Boil (leishmaniasis).

Notwithstanding this, I now knew who Carini was. But I felt an uncontrollable desire to know what he looked like. I wrote both Rio and São Paulo to obtain a photograph and even sent an emissary to Rio to find one (actually a fellow faculty member who was on his way there for a vacation). None of this was successful. Finally, the New York Academy of Medicine came through for me. Although they did not have a photograph on file, they keep records of where such photos might be obtained. In two papers dedicated to Carini's long and valued service in São Paulo, there appeared his likeness. He was a tiny, bald man, owl-eyed in dark tortoise shell rims, with a neatly clipped moustache and the flicker of a smile about his lips.

Thus it all finally fell into place as I have related to you in full. And now that I have satisfied my own curiosity about all this, I don't doubt that one or both of two questions might be raised in the mind of the reader. The first might be "How could a practicing cardiologist have the effrontery to take upon himself a task that would best be left in the hands of professional historians, especially those who have specialized in the history of infectious disease?" The second might be "How could anyone in his right mind expend so much time and effort on such a useless piece of medical minutia?" Let me deal with them in that order.

There is always a feeling of tension between amateurs who choose to delve into any kind of historical field and the professional historians who tend to bristle at the others' impertinence. I maintain that the only credentials one needs to write history are intelligence, self-discipline, honesty, and the ability to express oneself well in print. The latter, especially, is a precious quality too often missing in medical, historical, and other types of writing as well. One has only to read Winston Churchill or Barbara Tuchman, neither academically trained historians, to counter any objections. Churchill was a respected chronicler of world history as well as a maker of it. Throughout his life, he supported himself financially by such enterprises.

As for Tuchman, also self-trained, how much poorer the world would be without such works as *The Guns of August*, *Stillwell and the American Experience in China*, and especially, *A Distant Mirror*, her brilliant reconstruction of "the calamitous fourteenth century" in Europe. Chronically behind in my reading, I rarely open up a book a second time after I have finished it but find myself continually refingering the pages of her essays in *Practicing History* for guidance and inspiration.

Medicine has also had its literary lights. Recall that Harvey Cushing won a Pulitzer for his biography of William Osler. Then there is the elegant prose of Lewis Thomas, Richard Selzer, Oliver Sacks, Sherwin Nuland, and others who have won a wide and appreciative audience among medical and lay readers alike.

I should also like to point out that a disease can be likened to a crime. The patient is the victim and the cause of the disease the perpetrator. Professional historians can be looked upon as police investigators or emissaries from the district attorney's office, gathering clues to determine how well they can make a case. Doctors, nurses, and biological scientists are like relatives and close friends of the victim at the scene of the crime. Although unschooled in the formal rules of evidence, they can bring a sense of immediacy to their perception of the crime beyond that of any police officer or legal expert. It is for this reason that books such as Paul de Kruif's *The Microbe Hunters*, William Nolen's *The Making of a Surgeon* and *The Man Who Mistook His Wife for a Hat*, and other neurological tales by Oliver Sacks can have an impact unequalled by any professional medical historian, no matter how thorough or dedicated.

As for the apparent meaninglessness of my task, I must recall to you William Bennett Bean (1909–1989) who was frequently in my thoughts throughout the process. Dr. Bean was one of the last true *general* internists in the growing world of medical subspecialists. He could do very creditable research in cardiovascular disease and still be considered an expert in nutrition. He became interested in the skin manifestations of internal diseases and wrote a classic monograph on the subject, *Vascular Spiders and Related Diseases of the Skin*.[6] Toward the end of his life, he also completed a superb biography of Walter Reed,[7] and throughout the preceding years produced an unending flow of essays on subjects as diverse as herbals, Mrs. Henry Adams, Rabelais, Greek philosophy, Thomas Jefferson, John Shaw Billings, and Francis Bacon.

Bean's career in medicine was a peripatetic one, although he finally settled in at the University of Iowa College of Medicine where he chaired the department of medicine for over twenty years. Not surprisingly, few young physicians even recognize his name today. What is surprising, however, is the fact that although Bean authored over three hundred articles in his lifetime, among older physicians who remember him, it is his study on nail growth, his own, over installments spanning thirty-five years of sickness, health, aging, and changing climates and activity,[8] that sticks in their minds most vividly. Hardly the most serious of subjects for a serious investigator, but there it is.

A cynic has remarked that doctors write about medical history when they are no longer capable of making it. I see it differently. I think that the more experienced a physician becomes, the more at home he or she is with disease, the more it is possible to indulge the luxury of determining the finer points to fill in the little blanks about which we become "curiouser and curiouser." It enables us who live within the world of medicine to feel that the *terra* upon which we tread is just a bit more *cognita*. I have no doubts that Bean understood and appreciated the wonders of modern medicine, but he also emphasized another aspect of the art as he wrote about his observations on nail growth:

> The kind of pleasure and understanding that I get from studying natural history has long vanished from most of contemporary teaching institutions that have become part of intensive care units, which are supposed to save the residual intellectual machinery of medical students. . . . The capacity to look remains, but the capacity to see has all but vanished. Teachers and students forget that the ability to palpate is not the same as the ability to feel.

In tracking down Carini and his Pneumocystis, I believe now that unconsciously I was opening a door to this kind of intellectual experience. I certainly learned a bit about Carini, but I also learned much I did not know about parasitic diseases, the unpredictability of medical progress, and the capricious ways in which its achievements may or may not be rewarded. I also learned a good deal more about Chagas and his very important work, and something about Brazilian medical science as well.

And I was not about to stop. Tuberculosis is again on the rise, with not only AIDS patients at risk but those treating them and those living with them. The fact that resistant strains of tuberculosis are increasing as a medical problem underlines the importance of this new development. And then, for the umpteenth time I came upon the term "The White Plague" in reference to tuberculosis before I asked myself "Now where did this come from?" You won't believe what a merry chase this has led me. Ah, but that is another story.

Notes

1. Gajdusek DC. *Pneumocystis Carinii*—Etiologic agent of interstitial plasma cell pneumonia of premature and young infants. Pediatrics 1957; 19:543–565.

2. Kean BH. *MD: One Doctor's Adventures among the Famous and Infamous from the Jungles of Panama to a Park Avenue Practice.* New York: Random House, 1990.

3. Chagas C. Nova trypanosomiaza humana. Estudios sobre a morfologia e o ciclo evolutivo do *Schizotrypanum cruzi n. gen., n. sp.*, ajente etiologico de nova entidade morbida do homem. Mem Inst Oswaldo Cruz, Rio 1909; 1:159–217.

4. Delanoë P and Delanoë Mme. Sur les rapports des kysts de Carini du poumon des rats avec le *Trypanosoma lewisi.* CR Acad Sci 1912; 155:658–660.

5. Bacellar RC. *Brazil's Contributions to Tropical Medicine and Malaria.* Rio de Janeiro: Grafico Olimpica Editora, 1963.

6. Bean WB. *Vascular Spiders and Related Diseases of the Skin.* Springfield, Ill.: CC Thomas, 1958.

7. Bean WB. *Walter Reed: A Biography.* Charlottesville: Univ. Virginia Press, 1982.

8. Bean WB. Nail growth: Thirty-five years of observation. Arch Int Med 1980; 140:73–76.

5

Tuberculosis

Why "The White Plague"? (Another Detective Story)

THE IMPRINTS THAT diseases leave upon the societies they have descended upon are reflected in the various terms that have been applied to them historically. Tuberculosis, for example, has frequently been referred to as "The White Plague" in years past, although both components of that designation may be called into question.

To my way of thinking, tuberculosis has never constituted a plague, and ascribing whiteness to it also has raised serious doubts in my mind. According to *Webster's New Collegiate Dictionary*, a plague (from the Latin "to blow" or "strike") is "an epidemic disease causing a high rate of mortality: pestilence." Although this disease is traceable back to archaeological times, for the most important early descriptions of tuberculosis we must turn to the ancient Greeks, and it is unlikely that they ever considered it a plague in that sense. Rest assured they knew a plague when it hit them, the plague of Athens (430–426 B.C.) being the most famous. It claimed over 130,000 lives in a five-year period and included almost one-third of the city's foot soldiers and cavalrymen.

Hippocrates (460–370 B.C.) was alive in Greece during this plague but, fortunately for him, not located in that stricken city. Credited with one of the best early descriptions of tuberculosis, he and other Greeks of that period looked upon it quite differently from a plague. They used the term "phthisis" (Greek for decay or waste away) to describe its final manifestations. This emphasized the fact that although the rapidly progressive pulmonary form of the disease, which later came to be called "galloping consumption," could take off a victim in a relatively short time, many patients lived for a great number of years, sometimes as many as twenty or thirty, before succumbing. The terminal phase of phthisis, with extreme weight loss, was, at least in some patients, probably due to malabsorption of foodstuffs and diarrhea secondary to intestinal involvement that gave those dying of the disease their characteristic premortem appearance.

Even in the eighteenth and nineteenth centuries when tuberculosis was reported in the United States and parts of Western Europe to be the most common cause of death, the usual chronicity of the disease was well recognized. To use the term "plague" in reference to tuberculosis is obviously a misnomer.

What about "white"? The greatest currency given to the term in recent years might be ascribed to the use of "White Plague" as the title of the excellent book about the disease written by René Dubos and his second wife, Jean, and published in 1952.[1] René's first wife had died from the disease in 1942, and his second wife was afflicted with it during the time the book was being written. Inexplicably, nowhere in the book do the authors indicate the source of the term which they had chosen as its title. Selman Waksman (1888–1973), who was awarded a Nobel prize for his part in the introduction of streptomycin, the first effective medical therapy for the disease, in his own book about the disease, *The Conquest of Tuberculosis*,[2] mentions "white plague" three times, but again without revealing the source of the term. His codiscoverer, Albert Schatz, is still alive, but, when contacted by me in the course of this research, was unable to shed any further light on the origin of the term.

I wondered if the "white" in "white plague" related to race, pathology, the appearance of the patients, or perhaps some other aspect of the disease. Given the demographics of Western Europe and the United States, the popular use of the term might have been related to the preponderance of whites among their populations. However as it became evident that nonwhites were even more susceptible to the disease than whites and the proportion of whites continues to diminish among all these population groups, the ethnocentricity of the term is hardly justified.

What about the pathological appearance of the lesions? In Richard M. Burke's book *An Historical Chronology of Tuberculosis*,[3] mention is made of certain early postmortem descriptions. Included among them is Richard Wiseman's description of tuberculosis of the joints as "tumor albus" or white swelling (1676). Elsewhere I came across a description of the white tubercle of the liver. However, pulmonary tuberculosis is the most common form. As for the pulmonary tubercle, Matthew Baillie described it as gray in his early description (1793), and those who have followed him, including the great Laennec, have most often described the color as grayish or, following caseation, yellowish.

In terms of the patients' appearance, medical commentators over the last hundred years or more have often commented on the flushed appearance of the skin rather than pallor, at least early in the disease, this possibly related to their febrile state. Terminally, as the ancient Greeks had long ago emphasized, it is the extreme wasting of the patients that is noted invariably rather than any whiteness of complexion. Austin Flint (1812–1886) was considered an expert on tuberculosis and William Osler (1849–1919) an expert on everything. In Flint's textbook, published in 1886,[4] and the first edition of Osler's text, which appeared six years later,[5] no mention of "white plague" or white lesions in reference to tuberculosis are made, although in a multiauthored book on tuberculosis published in 1909, Osler in an historical introduction does use the term "white scourge" with no further comment on the term.[6]

Perhaps the world's last living authority on tuberculosis happened to be a colleague of mine at the New Jersey Medical School. The pathologist Oscar Auerbach, who had reached ninety-two at the time of his death in 1997 was, until the end, still active behind the microscope and making pertinently sage comments at morning medical report. During the 1930s and 1940s, he was pathologist at New York's Sea View Hospital on Staten Island, then probably the largest tuberculosis hospital in the world with its number of beds exceeding two thousand. During his time at Sea View, Auerbach performed over twenty-three hundred autopsies on patients dying from the disease and, among other contributions, clearly demonstrated that the body wasting of some patients, those with open cavities in the lung, was related to extensive involvement of the small intestine late in the disease. Diarrhea and lack of foodstuff absorption, present in over 70 percent of those in this category, accounted for the extreme malnutrition. Auerbach recalled to me that "You could lift them with a finger."

In the spring of 1994 during that conversation, Auerbach also recalled that in addition to the extreme cachexia, their extremely pale appearance was another terminal feature. This could have been accounted for by anemia. There can be blood loss in tuberculosis due to its expectoration following a breakdown in pulmonary vessels invaded by the disease process; if the intestines are involved, there may also be malabsorption of certain nutrients (e.g., B12) necessary for normal red blood cell formation. Finally, as in many chronic diseases, an otherwise unexplained anemia might occur. Auerbach remembered vividly the pallor of the white patients dying from the disease, but among the many nonwhites arriving at the morgue, this aspect of the terminal disease, he admitted, was not a prominent feature.

Unfortunately, Dr. Auerbach never performed any blood counts in his patients. However, Morris Braverman did. In 1938 he reported on "The Anaemia of Pulmonary Tuberculosis,"[7] pointing out that, while much work had been done on the white cell picture by previous investigators, "scant attention has been paid to the erythrocytes and anaemia." His findings revealed some degree of anemia, often not severe, in about one-third of the five hundred patients in whom blood counts had been performed as part of the autopsy procedure.

This paper appeared in the premiere tuberculosis journal in this country, The American Review of Tuberculosis (now The American Review of Respiratory Diseases), and was the first article on the subject of anemia in tuberculosis since the inception of the journal twenty-one years earlier. Obviously, the anemia of tuberculosis, such as it was, had not impressed many "phthisisists" over the years and hardly warranted the use of "white" in a popular term for the disease.

In summary then, it was clear that tuberculosis, despite its historical importance and growing threat in the age of AIDS, has never existed as a plague. And, with the growing awareness of its predominance among people of color, the pathological findings, as well as the absence of any evidence for severe anemia, the other half of the description handed down to us must also be seriously questioned.

Still, I felt a need to find out how and by whom the term had been introduced. As usual with this sort of quest, I began with the experts in the particular field involved, in this case the pulmonary and infectious disease physicians among my acquaintance. One of them seemed to remember a reference to Oliver Wendell Holmes (1809–1894), so I thought this would be a good place to start. Our librarian informed me that the New York Academy of Medicine had a complete collection of this distinguished Boston physician's writings, and I spent the better part of a day searching through them for a reference to tuberculosis. No luck.

However, my quest managed to infect one of the academy's history librarians with the same curiosity. He conducted an even more thorough search than mine but with no better result. So much for Holmes. But there were other promising sources beckoning. Within the first half of the current decade, three excellent books on tuberculosis had been published, and I immediately began searching them for references to "white plague" and contacting the authors for possible assistance.

In 1992 Barbara Bates's social history of the disease between 1876 and 1938 made no mention of the term.[8] When I called her, she drew a blank on the origin of the term "white plague" even though it was known to her. In the next year Frank Ryan's *The Forgotten Plague* was published. In it he had written, "From the seventeenth to the nineteenth century in England, like other great towns and cities [sic] in Europe and America it swept in a continuing epidemic of such monstrous proportions, the disease was called the White Plague of Europe."[9] A little hyperbolic, I thought, but as a student of the history of the disease, Ryan was certainly in a better position than I to comment upon it. I wrote and asked him about the source of "white plague," but he was unable to provide one. Nevertheless, he did raise the possibility that it was in Europe that I should be searching for the origin.

If this was the case, there was no better authority that I could consult than Arthur L. Bloomfield (1888–1962), who had been at Johns Hopkins and then chief of medicine at Stanford. He was a true scholar, whose intellectual roots were sunk deep into nineteenth as well as early-twentieth-century medicine. I believe he was fluent in French and German and probably well versed in Greek and Latin as well. It was unlikely that he had been ignorant of any of the important works on tuberculosis during this time in Europe as well as the United States. In 1958 he published a bibliography of communicable diseases in which he not only listed but summarized the findings of all the important publications related thereto.[10]

In regard to tuberculosis, I learned a good deal that would be surprising to any late-twentieth-century physician. For example, in 1826 as Laennec's second edition of lung and heart disease was being published and the author, himself, was dying from pulmonary tuberculosis at the age of forty-five, he and other physicians of the day were apparently unaware that the disease was contagious. Most thought it was related to certain constitutional and perhaps environmental factors. It was not until 1865 that another Frenchman, formerly unknown to me, J. A. Villemin, demonstrated that the disease was transmissible by implanting material from the lung of a recently dead patient to a rabbit.[11] He continued with such experiments, as did others, until finally Robert Koch identified the causative bacillus in 1882, with additional refinements in showing cause and transmission of infectious disease that later came to be called "Koch's postulates."[12] However, as for "white plague" there was nary a mention in Bloomfield's book.

My next best bet was Sheila M. Rothman of Columbia University whose 1994 book, *Living in the Shadow of Death*, focused on the history of the disease in the United States. Her feelings expressed about "white plague" were similar to my own ("in reality it [pulmonary tuberculosis] bore little resemblance to the epidemics that had earlier ravaged Europe").[13] I telephoned her to inquire about the origin of "white plague," and she offered the earliest source she had identified, a talk by Dr. Sigard Adolphus Knopf (1857–1940) to a medical society in St. Louis in 1904. Knopf had entitled the talk "The Possible Victory over the Great White Plague." I obtained a copy of the address, and among the opening remarks, the following statement is made: "From the title of my subject you know that I am to speak of tuberculosis as the 'Great White Plague.' "[14] Note the quotation marks.

Meanwhile the historian at the National Library of Medicine found an even earlier reference involving Knopf, a prize-winning essay he had submitted in 1899 to an international congress in Berlin about combating tuberculosis. Although there is no mention of white plague in the preface to the German edition of the essay, "Tuberculosis as a Disease of the Masses and How to Combat It," the preface to the American edition concludes "and let the people at large lend a willing hand in this combat against our common foe, the 'Great White Plague.' "[15] Again the term appears in quotes, suggesting another source. However, with no further leads to follow and with these two references to Knopf, both from reliable sources, I had to conclude that I had come to the end of the trail.

Who was Knopf? Born in Germany, he had immigrated to New York and by the turn of the century had become very active in the tuberculosis field, predominantly as a practitioner and proselytizer rather than a laboratory investigator. He was professor of physiotherapy at New York Post-Graduate Medical School and for over twenty years, a senior visiting physician at the Riverside Tuberculosis Hospital. Bed rest, fresh air, good diet, and improved sanitary conditions were the only means of treating tuberculosis in the pre-chemotherapy era, and undoubtedly in a number of cases, the disease was arrested if not cured. Knopf obviously considered it his mission to promote such measures to control the spread of the disease and effectively used the term "Great White Plague" to dramatize efforts toward this end.

End of story? Not quite. I continued to be troubled by Knopf's repeated use of quotation marks around the term, and I had the inescapable feeling that 1899 was still too recent. It was at this point that I recalled someone had mentioned an entry in the Random House unabridged English dictionary. I checked the entry; it read, "White plague: tuberculosis, esp. pulmonary, American 1865–1870."

I immediately called Random House in New York to determine if the source was possibly Oliver Wendell Holmes after all or someone else. They instructed me to fax the editor, Jesse T. Sheidlower, which I did, and within twenty-four hours, he had faxed back his reply.

> The attribution to O. W. Holmes is, to our knowledge, correct. . . . based on the following quotation from our files: "Two diseases especially have attracted attention above all others with reference to their causes and prevention; cholera, the "black death" of the nineteenth century, and consumption, the white plague of the north." (Oliver Wendell Holmes, *Medical Essays*, 1842–1882 [Boston, 2nd ed., 1892], 352)

Sheidlower assured me that I would be able to find this collection in our medical library, and indeed I did. How could I and the librarian at the New York Academy of Medicine have both missed it the first time around? Probably because the remark was buried in a lecture entitled "The Medical Profession in Massachusetts," delivered on January 29, 1869, before the Lowell Institute in Boston. It was obviously the title of the lecture and the inclusion of only a passing remark about tuberculosis that led to our error.

This hopefully final source of the term will probably put the question of origin to rest once and for all. In July 1994, our own history librarian entered our finding into "Caduceus" a national network of medical libraries, archivists, historians, and other interested parties to determine if anyone could come up with an earlier source. To date we have received no conflicting earlier reports.

Of course the question still remains as to precisely why Holmes called tuberculosis "white" (or cholera "black," for that matter). Given his present location, it is unlikely that either I or anyone else will ever be in a position to find out. However, if the true believers among us are correct, Dr. Holmes is looking down upon us and chuckling at our confusion. And some day in the not too near future, if I am lucky enough to wind up in the same place as Dr. Holmes, you may be sure that I will pop the question.

Notes

1. Dubos RJ and Dubos J. *"The White Plague" Tuberculosis: Man and Society*. Boston: Little Brown, 1952.
2. Waksman S. *The Conquest of Tuberculosis*. Berkeley: Univ. of California Press, 1964.
3. Burke RM. *An Historical Chronology of Tuberculosis*, 2nd ed. Springfield, Ill.: Thomas, 1955.
4. Flint A. *Treatise on the Principles and Practice of Medicine*, 6th ed. Philadelphia, Pa.: Lea Bros. & Co., 1886.
5. Osler W. *The Principles and Practice of Medicine*, 1st ed. New York: Appleton and Co., 1892.
6. Osler W. "Historical Sketch" in *Tuberculosis: A Treatise by American Authors on Its Etiology, Pathology, Frequency, Semeiology, Diagnosis, Prognosis, Prevention, and Treatment*. New York: Appleton, 1909.
7. Braverman M. The anaemia of pulmonary tuberculosis. Am Rev Tuberculosis 1938; 38:466–490.
8. Bates B. *Bargaining for Life: A Social History of Tuberculosis, 1876–1938*. Philadelphia: Univ. Pennsylvania Press, 1992.
9. Ryan F. *The Forgotten Plague: How the Battle Against Tuberculosis Was Won—and Lost*. Boston: Little Brown, 1993, 7.
10. Bloomfield AL. *A Bibliography of Internal Medicine: Communicable Diseases*. Chicago: Univ. Chicago Press, 1958.
11. Villemin JA. Cause et nature de la tuberculose. Bull Acad Med (Paris) 1865; 31:21.
12. Koch R. Die aetiologie der tuberculose. Berl Clin Wochnschr 1882; 19:221.
13. Rothman SM. *Living in the Shadow of Death: Tuberculosis and the Social Experience of Illness in America*. New York: Basic Books, 1994.
14. Knopf SA. The possible victory over the great white plague. St. Louis Courier of Medicine 1905; 32:129–142.
15. Knopf SA. *Tuberculosis as a Disease of the Masses and How to Combat It*. New York: Firestack, 1901.

6

Say It Isn't "No"

The Power of Positive Thinking in the Publication of Medical Research

HARVARD'S C. SIDNEY BURWELL is credited with the remark that half of what we teach our medical students will, in time, be shown to be wrong, but that, unfortunately, we do not know which half. To my knowledge, no one has ever seriously challenged that idea. If he was indeed right, logic would dictate that much of current medical research be devoted to correcting the fallacies of the past and that our journals be full of the re-search to set us straight.

Contrary to this expectation, however, I have often been struck, when perusing the medical literature, by the predominance of investigators with positive findings, with the naysayers in a distinct minority. On a personal level, my own studies that have challenged some previously reported data or beliefs have always had the most trouble getting published. Particularly galling about such rejections is the fact that those investigations were frequently the most difficult, tedious, and meticulously performed. It has seemed, at times, that the only way to get ahead in research was to be a perpetual yes-man.

In younger days I used to brood about this; as I grew older, I began to philosophize about it. What finally nudged these thoughts into print was the death a few years ago of Julius Comroe of the Cardiovascular Institute at the University of California in San Francisco. He was vitally interested in just how and why research is pursued, and certain of his writings should be required reading for anyone interested in doing scientific investigation.[1]

In an address he once made to a meeting of cardiologists, Dr. Comroe, tongue-in-cheek, confessed that he had once committed a grievous error in his own research career. He had attempted to repeat a previously successful experiment—and failed.

Before committing myself to a grievous error in print, I felt obliged to attempt some verification of my impression about the power of positive research and the difficulties in gaining an audience for negative results. There have been studies on the types of medical research performed, the changing productivity of investigators, the ethics of human research, and even the number of authors of papers published over the years, but I could not find studies about negative research. The *Index Medicus* does not even include the term, and a MEDLARS (Medical Literature Analysis and Retrieval System) search for it under various guises proved fruitless.

An examination of this question was certainly in order, and a few years back I began with a good general medical journal, the *New England Journal of Medicine*. I reviewed all the original articles published in the calendar year 1984 and classified them according to the conclusions reached as having positive findings, negative results, or neither (neutral studies on the basis of inconclusive or mixed results). I excluded articles with fewer than five subjects, those of a nature inapplicable to the planned categorization, and those I simply could not understand. Since the purpose of my survey was merely to confirm or refute a personal impression and not to convince any corps of statisticians that might be lying in wait for me at some editorial office, I attempted no formal evaluations of statistical significance—I refused to be undone by a p value.

I reviewed 208 articles. Of these, 168 were positive in their conclusions, 20 negative, and 20 neutral (80 percent, 10 percent, and 10 percent respectively). Did that low number of negative studies, given the Burwell dictum, indicate anything idiosyncratic about the *New England Journal of Medicine*? To check on this, I reviewed the first one hundred papers in the *Annals of Internal Medicine* for the same year: 89 percent positive, 1 percent negative, 10 percent neutral. The results of a similar analysis in the *Annals of Surgery*: 91 percent positive, 3 percent negative, 6 percent neutral.

At one point it had occurred to me that perhaps there might be more room for admission of doubt among the abstracts presented at a medical meeting. After all, they all would not automatically become part of the medical literature. Over a year's time after the presentation of such papers at these meetings, less than half the abstracts may actually result in permanent publications.[2] Of one hundred presented papers randomly selected from the 1984 meeting of the American Federation for Clinical Research, 95 percent turned out to be positive, 2 percent negative, and 3 percent neutral. One must conclude that it pays to be positive.

As for the reverse, the bad news bearers of medical research have never fared well. This is something of a mystery, especially when one recalls how often we have been victimized by our collective overenthusiasm and gullibility.

The flub of the century in this context is often laid at the door of Professor Johannes Fibiger, the Danish pathologist who first found worms in the stomach cancers of rats in 1907. He later mistakenly concluded that the worms caused the cancer. By the time 1913 rolled around, he had reported his work on the experimental induction of Spiroptera carcinoma in rodents.[3] In 1926 he was awarded the Nobel Prize in Physiology and Medicine. Meanwhile, Peyton Rous at the Rockefeller Institute, who was really on to something in 1910 when he demonstrated the transfer of chicken sarcomas with a cell-free filtrate,[4] was virtually ignored for his contribution to understanding the association between viruses in cancer. In 1966, after more than half a century and more than twenty nominations, Rous, then eighty-seven, finally received his just recognition in Stockholm.

Whatever the error of his work, Fibiger did not mean to mislead us. But there were mental aberrants who were just as successful in leading the scientific community astray. Cyril Burt, the English psychologist who dominated the field in the 1930s and 1940s, and whose work on separated identical twins was critical to the position of those who believed in the primacy of inherited intelligence, manufactured not only twin pairs out of thin air, but collaborators as well. John Darsee, the promising cardiologist whose faked research at both Emory and Harvard was finally uncovered in 1981, mixed up valid studies with his fabricated data, which may have provided him with something of a smokescreen. But why were those men so successful for so long? There certainly were many critical minds in England and the United States. Although many factors can be implicated, the simple desire of all around them to glow in the reflection of all those lovely positive results must have been a major consideration—as one gathers from reading the interviews with those concerned.

Still, whatever the source of the misinformation involved, it is a comfort to realize that sometime, somewhere there will be someone who will take a very close look. Fortunately, there are those among us who have an almost unreasonable persistence in pursuing their hunches even when previous evidence is to the contrary. There are also those with a persnickety compulsion to prove to themselves that what others have found is really correct. It is they who are the heroes of this piece.

Perhaps it was just such compulsion that prompted J. H. Tijo and A. Levan, thirty-three years after the number of human chromosomes had been established as forty-eight, to do a recount and find, with newer techniques, that it was really forty-six.[5] That kind of thinking was surely instrumental in motivating George Cotzias and his associates to pursue their work with levodopa in the treatment of parkinsonism when others had reported failures and unacceptable side effects.[6]

It took decades for the moment of truth to emerge, but through his own statistical analyses, Princeton's Leon Kamin uncovered the forgeries of Cyril Burt.[7] Fraud revealed can even have a bright side. It was the failure of others at Sloan-Kettering and in other institutions to repeat William Summerlin's experiments with mouse-skin transplantation that set the search for explanations in motion. Summerlin, unable to repeat his transplants successfully after his transfer from Minnesota to New York, was pressured by criticism into finally presenting his superior, Robert Good, with the now famous painted mice. But in the aftermath of the scandal it was found that in coming to New York, Summerlin had unconsciously altered the conditions of the experiment. Those alterations might well have been the reason for the failure to reproduce the original experimental results.

Such dramatic episodes underline the importance of reassessing the body of medical knowledge. What they do not tell us is how much of that body needs to be reassessed. Holes can easily be poked in the analysis I have undertaken here. Many of the articles printed are not really the results of experiments but simply descriptive or epidemiologic that should not fall into the categories discussed here. Another type of report, a new test for something that had failed in the originator's laboratory, certainly has no place in cluttering up the literature. So all reports of new laboratory tests would naturally be positive.

When it was decided to include this essay, written about ten years ago, as part of the current collection, another consideration presented itself. Could times have changed? Had the inclinations of authors or editors altered over the last decade? This prompted a revisit to the *New England Journal of Medicine*, this time to look at the volumes for 1995. Perhaps the practices or format of the journal had changed, or perhaps its contributors, or perhaps my own criteria for selection, but this time around, I could only cull about half the number of articles (107) meeting the same criteria for selection used a decade earlier.

Nevertheless, the breakdown was just about the same: 78 percent positive, 11 percent negative, and 11 percent neutral.

One final question might be asked: "Was Burwell really wrong in the first place?"

Could it be that there is *not* that large amount of false information lying about awaiting correction? Could this then account for the paucity of negative reports in the literature? Back in 1986 I had taken another look at the *New England Journal of Medicine* articles reviewed, hoping to find a clue. Which articles actually examined previous research or current practices?

Among the 208 articles, I had found that 37 could be classified in that category. Of these, 18 confirmed the earlier work, 10 challenged it, and 9 were inconclusive. With the 1995 review, I found 11 articles of this type, 5 confirming the previous work, and 6 refuting it. Burwell did say that half of what we teach our medical students will, in time, be shown to be wrong. From this sample it appears that Burwell was very close to the mark if not right on it. One might even suspect that at least some editors are not all that prone to "accentuate the positive/eliminate the negative." But I would like to keep the book open on that one.

Notes

1. Comroe JH Jr and Dripps RD. Ben Franklin and open heart surgery. Circ Res 1974; 35:661; Comroe JH Jr. *Retrospectroscope: Insights into Medical Discovery*. Menlo Park, Calif.: Von Gehr Press, 1977.

2. Goldman L and Loscalzo A. Fate of cardiology research originally published in abstract form. New Engl J Med 1980; 303:255.

3. Fibiger J. Recherches sur un nématode et sur sa faculté de provoquer des néoformations papillomateuses et carcinomateuses dans l'estomac du rat. Académie Royale des Sciences et des Lettres de Danemark. 1913.

4. Rous P. A sarcoma of the fowl transmissible by an agent separable from the tumor cells. J Exp Med 1911; 13:397.

5. Tijo JH and Levan A. The chromosome number in man. Hereditas 1956; 42:1–6.

6. Cotzias GC, Van Woert MH, Schiffer LM. Aromatic amino acids and modification of parkinsonism. N Engl J Med 1967; 276:374.

7. Kamin LJ. *The Science and Politics of IQ*. Potomac, Md.: Erlbaum Assoc., 1974.

7

Beyond the Bench

A Vote for Clinical Research

THE REMARK WAS made at a meeting of the senior faculty of our Department of Medicine not long ago. An upcoming vote involved awarding a tenured position to a candidate whose qualifications did not seem quite up to the mark to some of those present. The frustrated proposer of the appointment slammed a fist on the table.

"Dammit, this man's a true scientist, not just another clinical investigator."

This seemed a little odd, at a time when so many are deploring the lack of good clinical investigators. Having performed both basic science and clinical research during my own professional life, at times simultaneously, I began to think about this dichotomy.

I suppose the big dividing line is people. The clinical investigator deals largely with patients, whereas the "true scientist" remains behind the closed doors of his lab. Certainly, the laboratory worker is most highly esteemed within the scientific community. If you doubt it, just take a look at the winners of the Nobel Prize in Medicine and Physiology for the past two decades. It is clear that anyone working at the macromolecular level is at a distinct disadvantage when medicine's most prestigious awards are handed out.

There is something esthetically pristine about the work of the bench scientist, hidden away among his mice, flasks, test tubes, and other laboratory paraphernalia. In such a milieu, there is a great opportunity for individual expression—and later, individual recognition. The basic scientist is autonomous in his or her domain, having no superimposed protocol. Reading *The Double Helix*, for example, one has the distinct impression of a conspiratorial collaboration between James D. Watson and Francis Crick in their successful attempt at divining the structure of DNA.

But you cannot quietly go your own way in conducting human (i.e., clinical) research when there is the need to ensure that the patients or volunteers are fully informed and protected. As for individuality, it is often lost. Participation as just one of a team in a large multicenter study is often the fate of clinical investigators. And yet, granting the primary importance of basic research, the two must work hand in hand to benefit society. For example, what use would all our basic knowledge about the polio and hepatitis viruses have been without the large clinical trials that proved the efficacy of vaccines to prevent such infections? The basic scientist is truly the architect of the temple of medicine, whereas the clinical researchers provide the brick and mortar.

In addition to the opportunity for individual expression afforded by laboratory research, another aspect is generally unappreciated by the public. A sense of playfulness can be brought to bear when one's work is performed so close to the chest, as this story, perhaps apocryphal, illustrates. At the end of a long day of meaningless results, so the tale goes, a couple of researchers decided to relieve their boredom and exasperation by relieving *themselves* into the uncooperative brew that was about to be discarded. To their surprise and delight, some early data about urokinase, an important dissolver of blood clots, resulted from this frivolous act of frustration.

It is difficult to imagine a similar scenario in a multicenter study involving human investigation. Yet, it is possible to add some spice in ferreting out information about humans, simply by the selection of unusually promising segments of the population. This has certainly been done in cardiovascular research.

One of my earliest recollections is of a study done by J. N. Morris nearly forty years ago. It involved sedentary London bus drivers and their scurrying fare collectors and demonstrated an increase in coronary disease among the former compared to the latter. Although flawed in several respects, it started us thinking about the role of physical activity, or the lack of it, in the pathogenesis of coronary heart disease. Later on, a counting of heads among Harvard alumni provided another clue to the apparent protectiveness of regular exercise vis-à-vis coronary heart disease.

What of other aspects of life style? Coronary heart disease was once looked upon as a disease of the rich and powerful, those at the top of the societal heap. Yet, it turns out that the higher echelons of corporate structure are not at the highest risk nor is the labor force at the bottom—but rather the supervisory personnel who are squeezed in between. We learned that better, or at least higher, education gave something of a protective edge in this arena. And that if you happened to be a monk, you were much better off as a Trappist than as a Benedictine. (The answer lay in the fat content of their diets.)

One of the most interesting—albeit controversial—clinical investigations of heart disease was Dr. Meyer Friedman's classification of the striving, time-pressured type A and the more "laid back" type B personalities. There is less disagreement about more tangible factors: cigarette smoking, hypertension, and the importance of blood lipid levels.

Ancel Keys and his associates put an old adage to the test: You are what you eat (or at least your coronaries are). This culminated in the landmark seven-country study that appeared in 1970 and, with additional population studies by Keys and others, was an important stimulus to dietary modification among coronary-prone men. Groups as disparate as the African Masai and Seventh-day Adventists have since been subjected to the investigative probes of such researchers.

Improved gadgetry has provided other eye-opening chapters in the clinical investigation of heart disease, evaluating the effects of physiologic stress. Electrocardiographic monitoring of the patient with an acute myocardial infarction was extended to the patient's bed at home, and after weeks of observation, attempts were made to define the optimal coital position for post-coronary patients. We have hooked up many others thanks to Holter monitoring. The arrhythmogenic potential of hotly contested basketball or football games was clearly demonstrated when coaches submitted to wiring. House staff on morning rounds were not immune to similar electrical instability when embarrassing questions were asked.

Echocardiography provided new vistas to selected segments of our society: dancers, marathon runners, weight lifters, and others, showing that "normal" for these groups might be different from that for the rest of us.

In all of these applications of clinical research, the findings could be fairly well understood by our subjects, and their cooperation was forthcoming in the interest of their own well-being.

Something else started me down this cardiovascular memory lane: an abstract I came upon before attending the annual meeting of the American College of Cardiology not long ago. As I scanned the abstracts of the program with its seemingly endless listing of superscientific but often repetitive and even soporific abstruse titles, I came across a beaut: "Circadian Pattern of Heart Rate Is Altered by Stress: Study of Continuous Electrocardiographic Monitoring During Strauss, Mozart, Rachmaninoff, and Tchaikovsky."

We know that our heart rates normally peak during the early morning hours and then gradually decline, with a low point reached at night. D. Mulcahy and his associates at the National Heart Hospital and the Occupational Health Department of the British Broadcasting System in London wanted to assess the effects of different temporal patterns of work on this pattern.

They monitored forty-seven members of the BBC Symphony Orchestra over twenty-four-hour periods, including final rehearsals and live evening performances. They found that the primary peak in heart rate was in the evening rather than early morning, where a secondary lower peak persisted. To prove that it was not only the playing of instruments that caused this, they demonstrated a similar pattern among the five members of the management-technical team who were monitored simultaneously.

But the most intriguing piece of information (for me) was missing. What was the effect on the audience? And was there a difference between Mozart and Strauss? And which Strauss, Johann from Vienna or Richard from Bavaria?

I chuckled, recalling a somewhat off-color joke about two brothers, one good and one bad, who were suddenly killed in an auto accident. The good one goes to heaven, where he is bored to tears by the blandness of the place, with the heavenly choir providing a sort of Muzak backdrop. He peers over the side of his heavenly perch and sees his brother in a snug corner of Hades with a bottle of wine in one hand, a beautiful blonde on his lap, and the best hi-fi equipment installed all about him. The good brother visits his wayward sibling to complain about the injustice of it all but is quickly assured that it really *is* hell down there. The bottle happens to have a hole in the bottom, the blonde does not, and the music is all Bartok!

What, one wonders, might have been the contrasting effects of Mozart versus Bartok on circadian rhythms? And how about Stravinsky? Recall that the premiere of *The Rite of Spring* resulted in a near riot in the Paris of 1913. Now *that* would have been a study!

However, I was fated never even to ask the question, because the abstract somehow disappeared from the final program, and the paper was never read. Perhaps contemplation of the adverse effects this presentation might have had on his own circadian rhythm dissuaded the author from going through with it. Or perhaps the program committee, in a moment of serious reflection, decided that it would have proved to be just too much fun, or maybe just too—ugh—clinical.

8

Mostly about Books—and Medicine

HERE IS A typical New York story: my father's employer, a well-educated and wealthy clothing manufacturer, lived on West Eighty-first Street directly across from the American Museum of Natural History. He lived there for over twenty years. Not once in all that time did he ever venture a foot inside that incredible repository of knowledge and experience. Here is another: born and bred in New York City and having lived almost all my life within an hour's travel from Forty-second Street and Fifth Avenue, I was past sixty when, for the first time, I crossed the threshold of the main branch of the New York Public Library, another hallowed center of learning within the great city.

Even then, it was not on my own account that I visited that august institution; I was simply searching within for my son who had, himself, gone there only to look up a reference for his girlfriend who was then living in Boston. (I must admit some sense of embarrassment at this confession.)

Once inside, I experienced a feeling of elation. For, as I wandered about the vast and stately halls and reading rooms, I was overwhelmed by an aura of sanctity in the place and even more by the activity within. There I saw men and women of all ages intently pouring through all kinds of reading material, making notes, soaking up information and even seeming to enjoy it—in a very serious sort of way, of course.

We are supposed to be living in an age when "the medium is the message" (whatever that means!) and when data storage banks, computers, and TV screens will perform the same sorts of tasks that conventional libraries and books once did, and ever so much better. But here I saw for myself the sense of satisfaction and, in some cases, perhaps even exhilaration that comes from holding a book within one's hands and absorbing all it has to offer.

Although I like to think of myself as a scholarly sort of person, I would hardly characterize myself as being bookish. I indulge a passion for history—political as well as scientific—but fiction of all kinds generally leaves me cold. I rarely buy a book for the mere pleasure of reading it once. If I do not intend to use it as a reference source, it has a hard time earning a place on my bookshelf. So why all this excitement about books?

I believe that for me, as well as for many other physicians, it was the reading of one book or perhaps several that proved a turning point in our lives, heading us toward a career in medicine. Albert Sabin of polio fame tells the story of his own conversion. It happened after reading Paul de Kruif's *Microbe Hunters* while he was still a dental student at New York University. Many of us, much less distinguished than this great microbiologist, must have similar stories to tell, I thought. But how many? What books? And to what extent do such considerations affect the current crop of physicians in the making?

Back in 1992 in order to satisfy my initial curiosity about premed students' reading habits prior to applying to medical school, I devised a one page questionnaire and asked a class of freshman at the New Jersey Medical School (NJMS) to fill it out. I included some space for other information for correlation, with the names of those queried omitted to permit a greater freedom of response. A lecturer in anatomy was kind enough to provide me with ten minutes of his hour to do the deed, and another colleague volunteered to help with statistical analysis.

For a comparative sampling elsewhere, I first considered sending the questionnaire to geographically contrasting classes of freshmen: in New England, the South, or the Midwest, perhaps. But then a more intriguing matchup came to mind. My own group, the class of 1958 from Downstate in Brooklyn, was about to celebrate its thirty-fifth year since graduation. What an opportunity to compare the changing faces and fashions in premedical reading habits over three and a half decades!

The Downstate Class of 1958, as I reviewed it in our graduation yearbook, and the New Jersey Medical School class of 1996 had interesting similarities as well as differences. Both schools are situated in industrialized, densely populated northeastern states. Both are state schools with large class sizes and are part of a statewide system of medical education (The State University of New York, SUNY, and the University of Medicine and Dentistry of New Jersey, UMDNJ). Finally there was even a sizable contingent of New Jersey residents admitted to Downstate in 1954 because at that time there were no operating medical schools in New Jersey and an interstate agreement provided for such an admissions policy. (The Seton Hall School of Medicine, which later became the New Jersey Medical School, would not open its doors in Jersey City until 1956.)

Table 8.1 Comparison of the Classes of 1958 and 1996 (%)

	Class of 1958 (N = 146)	Class of 1996 (N = 154)
Sex		
Male	92	51
Female	8	49
Race		
White	98	49
African-American	1	9
Hispanic/Latino	0	10
Asian-American	1	25
Unstated	0	7
M.D. relatives[a]		
None	73	66
One or more	27	34
Family income[a]		
Low	51	8
Average	34	41
Above average	15	41
High	0	10
"Readers"[a]	28	31

[a] For the class of 1958, information obtained from 61 respondents to questionnaire.

Although there were these similarities, they were dramatically overshadowed by the differences. As indicated in Table 8.1, the Downstate Class of 1958 was almost exclusively white (98 percent) and male (92 percent). Most striking to me, in retrospect over thirty years later, was the fact that over 70 percent of the 146 graduates were Jewish. This was not totally out of line, given New York City's ethnic mix and the large number of Jewish undergraduates emanating from its colleges. However, it is noteworthy in another respect: it was a sign that the years of medical school exclusionary practices based on religious quotas had been coming to an end. The record regarding other minorities was, frankly, scandalous yet representative of medical schools in general back then. There were only two blacks, one man of Chinese ancestry, and no Hispanics. Also characteristic of the time, women accounted for less than 10 percent of the whole graduating class.

In marked contrast to this, within the NJMS freshman class of 154 students, almost half of its members were women. Blacks and Hispanics/Latinos are significantly represented; but most impressive, I thought, is the number of Asian-Americans (of whom about half were of Indian background).

To obtain additional information regarding the Class of 1958 for this project, I devised a questionnaire similar to that presented to the current freshman medical students, and sent it to the 130 surviving members whose addresses were known to our Alumni Association. Sixty-one, including me, replied.

The lower half of Table 8.1 shows this additional comparative data. Interestingly the connection with medical relatives (e.g., fathers, mothers, uncles, aunts, etc.) was similar when the two groups were compared. However, while over half of the Downstaters responded that their family income at the time they entered medical school was low, only few of the NJMS freshmen claimed familial poverty ($p < 0.001$). Among my classmates, 28 percent claimed that their career choice had been influenced by their reading (we will call them "readers" as distinguished from "nonreaders" for the sake of convenience here) and a similar proportion for this, 31 percent, for the NJMS Class of 1996.

There was one surprise in store for me: although the number of women in my own class was too small to make comparisons, among the "readers" at the NJMS, the ratio of men to women among the readers was 1.7/1.0. The difference was not statistically significant ($p < 0.07$), but still it impressed me because I had expected to find a preponderance of women among the readers.

What were the books that influenced the two classes of medical students, separated by a span of thirty-five years or so?

The most popular choices of the seventeen readers reporting from my own class (including me) are indicated in Table 8.2. I had been "turned on" to medicine by de Kruif's book as well as by Hans Zinsser's *Rats, Lice, and History*, which dwelt on the effects of infectious diseases, especially typhus, on world history. Haggard's *Devils, Drugs, and Doctors* was another favorite of mine along with Victor Heiser's stories about his medical travels in the Far East as recounted in *An American Doctor's Odyssey*. Books about our growing knowledge and ability to control infectious diseases were popular for my generation in view of the major advances that had preceded it and the still predominant role they had to play in the mortality figures of our society in preceding years. Hans Zinsser expressed it best in the first chapter of his own book in which he wrote, "Infectious disease is one of the few genuine adventures left in the world."[1] His and Haggard's writing still stand up well today while the gee-

Table 8.2 Most Popular Influential Books Selected by the Class of 1958 (N = 17)

Title	Number
Nonfiction	
Microbe Hunters (P. de Kruif, 1926)	8
Devils, Drugs, and Doctors (Howard H. Haggard, 1929)	2
Rats, Lice, and History (Hans Zinsser, 1935)	2
The Doctors Mayo (H. Clapesattle, 1941)	2
Fiction	
Arrowsmith (Sinclair Lewis, 1925)	6

Table 8.3 Most Popular Influential Books Selected by the Class of 1996 (N = 48)

Title	Number
Nonfiction	
Love, Medicine, and Miracles (Bernie S. Siegel, 1986)	5
The House of God (Samuel Shem, 1978)	4
Becoming a Doctor (Melvin Konner, 1987)	4
Gifted Hands (Benjamin S. Carson, 1990)	3
M.D.: Doctors Talk about Themselves (John Pekannen, 1988)	3
A Taste of My Own Medicine (Edward Rosenbaum, 1988)	3
Fiction	
Doctors (Erich Segal, 1989)	4
The Citadel (A. J. Cronin, 1937)	3

whiz-gosh-golly style that characterized the even more popular *Microbe Hunters* seems a bit passé.

Other nonfiction reported from my class included the writings of Freud, and biographies of Pasteur, cardiologist James B. Herrick and Elizabeth Blackwell, the first woman to graduate from an American medical school. Among the books of fiction, Sinclair Lewis's *Arrowsmith* was far and away the most popular, no doubt abetted by de Kruif's assistance behind the scenes. Waltari's *The Egyptian* and Norton Thompson's *Not As a Stranger* also received honorable mention.

Table 8.3 lists the most popular choices of the NJMS Class of 1996. Not surprisingly there appear newer books about medicine (alas, none of my own) compared to the most influential ones affecting my own generation, books published between 1924 and 1942. On reviewing the nonfiction entries of our current freshmen, I was impressed by the curious amalgam of naïveté and cynicism reflected in their choices. At the top of the list, Bernie Siegel's feel good philosophy of medicine seemed to prevail, while at the cynical end of the scale were books with titles such as *In Sickness and in Wealth*, *Doctor Cool*, *A Not Entirely Benign Procedure*, and *Year of the Intern*. However, as may be seen from the table, many excellent books about medicine were also included, with mention also made of Lewis Thomas, Oliver Sacks, and a few others not in the top ranking. A half dozen textbooks were entered, ranging from general science to birth defects in subject matter.

Their fiction list had another one of my nonfavorites at the top, Erich Segal, but I was pleased to see A. J. Cronin's *The Citadel* still in the running, with his *Shannon's Way* a single entry with other works from Camus, Mann, Dickens, Solzhenitsyn, John Irving, and Michael Crichton.

The Holy Bible was mentioned twice.

So there it is. And, despite the generational disparities in taste, one can take some comfort in the knowledge that, even in this age of TV bites and computer bits, young people can still find pleasure by curling up with a good book of their choice—and it might even make a difference in their lives.

Note

1. Zinsser H. *Rats, Lice, and History*. Boston: Back Bay Books, Little, Brown and Co., 1965, 13.

9

Confessions of Creeping Obsolescence

THE MEMORY OF James B. Herrick (1861–1954) is revered by hematologists and cardiologists alike. He was considered to be one of their own by both groups of specialists. In 1910, it was Herrick who first described those peculiarly shaped red blood corpuscles characteristic of sickle cell anemia.[1] Two years later, in another landmark paper, he pointed out that sudden obstruction of a coronary artery did not always result in immediate death.[2] Herrick acknowledged that he was not the first to recognize the clinical features of what we now call acute myocardial infarction and, indeed, quoted the writings of others to support his own arguments about nonlethal coronary occlusions. However, Herrick's report undoubtedly had the most influence in spreading the word and leading future physicians toward better recognition, treatment, and prevention of coronary heart disease.

Given the period during which Herrick reached his medical maturity, it is highly unlikely that he ever considered himself a hematologist or cardiologist. Even to have called him an internist would have been premature. "Internists," got their start in Germany during the early 1880s, but the designation arrived here a good deal later. It was not until 1945 that the American Medical Association actually replaced "the practice of medicine" with "internal medicine."[3]

Although he founded the Society of Internal Medicine of Chicago in 1915, Herrick, in his prime, would have most likely been simply called a physician (or possibly a consultant) with a particular interest in matters involving the cardiovascular and hematologic systems. Whatever one calls him, Herrick, for all his accomplishments and success, was prey to the lifelong affliction of all internists: the difficulty of keeping up with such a massive and all-encompassing field. So concerned was he about his ignorance of chemistry, which was coming to dominate medical thought and research at the beginning of the century, that he temporarily abandoned a busy private practice in 1904 at the age of forty-three in order to update his knowledge. The process included a trip to Germany for further training in this discipline.

Even the patron saint of internal medicine, Sir William Osler, was not immune to pangs of inadequacy. In his memoirs, Herrick recalls a meeting with Osler at an AMA convention in 1902 when, confronted with an array of biochemical representations placed on the blackboard by some speaker, Osler expressed the longing to be nineteen again and able to "do it all over."[4] Whatever his misgivings about the state of his knowledge, Osler had not been deterred from writing a textbook of medicine a decade earlier—and a darned good one at that. Given the continued expansion of our specialty, who among us would have the temerity to attempt a similar feat today? Who would even attempt a monograph on a subspecialty without the assistance of super specialists within the field?

As a cardiologist, I have always liked to think of myself as an internist first. As such, I have accepted that chronic anxiety about keeping up that comes with the territory, but it has not been easy. The seeds of my own self-doubt were already sown by the time I had left medical school. Sir Hans A. Krebs was primarily responsible.

Practically our entire course in biochemistry was devoted to the elucidation of the citric acid cycle, for which Krebs, incidentally, with Fritz A. Lipmann was awarded a Nobel Prize in Physiology and Medicine in 1953. At each lecture our professor would chalk up another segment of the saga until at the final session, the whole thing appeared on blackboards lining the large lecture hall, and our professor, unwittingly in deference to Krebs's Teutonic origins, had drawn all the leitmotivs together in a Gotterdammerung-like exposition.

In more than thirty-five years of medical practice, I have yet to bring the Krebs cycle to the bedside, for all its importance and brilliance.

It was not only biochemistry. Take hematology as another example of my growing ineptitude. Somewhere back in the dim past, the clotting scheme was as delightfully comprehensible as it was incomplete. Prothrombin-to-thrombin-to-fibrin had a Tinker-to-Evers-to-Chance simplicity that was 100 percent American in some way. But even when I was a medical student in the late 1950s, those Roman numbered clotting factors were beginning to clutter up the picture: Factor V, VII, IX, and X were almost familiar to me by the time I graduated in 1958. But new ones kept on coming. And to further complicate the picture, for every new clotting factor there seemed to be an associated anticlotting factor. "Cascade" is the name they now give to the clotting process, and I have nightmarish visions of factor MDCCXVII and all of its predecessors engulfing me in a monstrous lava-like flow of hemic ooze. All this without even getting into the tissue factors involved.

The variety of white blood cells also seems to be expanding exponentially. It is no longer adequate to define them on the basis of their morphology or staining properties. Each new type is now categorized on the basis of its personality. It is either a killer cell or a helper cell or some other type of well-adjusted or malevolent character.

It is just as bad with prostaglandins. Ever since Ulf von Euler got the ball rolling in the 1930s, they seem to have appeared in almost every organ system. But in medical practice they remain at a distance, like some highly respected foreign guests with whom, because of the language barrier, we cannot adequately communicate.

Henderson-Hasselbalch is to acid-base balance what wheat is to bread, but my only contribution in practice is to primly correct the medical student who inadvertently omits the second "l" in Hasselbalch. It is true that I now find the "anion gap" not totally confusing and am even able to calculate it on occasion despite the persistent gaps, I am sure, in my understanding.

Arthur Kornberg once sent me a reprint of his paper entitled "For the Love of Enzymes." He even used this as the title for his autobiography.[5] Loving enzymes was a bit much for me, but I have tried my level best at least to like them. Unfortunately, I must confess that they simply don't seem to like me.

Infectious disease is another source of dismay for the internist who would like to keep abreast of recent developments. Long ago, however, I gave up on this as well. As a self-respecting cardiologist and busy echocardiographer, I take second place to no one in estimating my abilities to diagnose infective endocarditis. But once the diagnosis is made, I despair of selecting the right antibiotic or recommended combination of the day or week, and turn the decision over to my infectious disease colleagues. There is too much danger of selecting a third generation cephalosporin when only a fourth will do—or are we already on to the fifth or sixth?

And so it goes through every province of the vast realm we call internal medicine: gastroenterology, immunology, endocrinology, rheumatology, and the rest. This does not mean that, as a cardiologist, I do not have my own areas of esoterica with which to confuse other internists. In the past we cardiologists could dazzle by juggling several different kinds of digitalis preparation. Then we developed our classification of antiarrhythmics. Now we can befuddle our confreres with a bewildering array of beta blockers, calcium channel blockers, and ACE inhibitors. But this only serves to emphasize the hopelessness of effort in the entire body of practicing internists.

And yet, quixotically, I persist. I once counted the number of journals I read or scan. An incomplete list includes five general medical journals, four internal medicine journals, ten cardiovascular journals, two basic science journals in cardiovascular physiology, and three scientific journals with broader scope, not to mention the *New York Times*. I am not sure how much they have helped.

The late Sir George Pickering, Regius Professor of Medicine at Oxford, was noted for his work on hypertension, but he was no slouch on problems concerned with learning the new medicine and doing away with the old. He also had a devilishly witty way of putting things. In a slim volume containing his views on medical education, he dispensed with the old fogies of medicine as follows: "Where there is death there is hope."[6]

As the intellectual deadwood within the medical community gets removed, our students, who did their medical teething on rings of recombinant DNA, will undoubtedly be less confused by what is new in medicine, and this, I suppose, is how progress is made. In the meantime, the rest of us will continue to live with our doubts about our ability to fulfill our early hopes and expectations.

But there is some solace to be found in this dilemma. It is just such insecurity about the extent of our knowledge that spurs us on to continued self-education. Because of our concern about being able to do right by our patients, we try that much harder—and perhaps the care we provide might even be just a little bit better.

Notes

1. Herrick JB. Peculiar elongated and sickle-shaped red blood corpuscles in a case of severe anemia. Trans Assoc Am Phys 1910; 25:553.
2. Herrick JB. Clinical features of sudden obstruction of the coronary arteries. JAMA 1912; 59:2015.
3. Bean WB. Origin of the term "internal medicine." New Engl J Med 1982; 306:182.
4. Herrick JB. *Memories of Eighty Years*. Chicago: Univ. Chicago Press, 1949.
5. Kornberg A. *For the Love of Enzymes*. Boston: Harvard Univ. Press, 1989.
6. Pickering G. *Quest for Excellence in Medical Education*. Oxford: Oxford Univ. Press, 1978, 44.

10

Man's Best Friend

I KILLED MY last dog in 1982. In the papers we published we ordinarily referred to this act as one of "sacrifice." Call it a euphemism or simply a more meaningful description. I don't believe any of our dogs were capable of making such fine distinctions.

During the first twenty years of my efforts at cardiovascular research, I probably disposed of hundreds of dogs. I did not stop because of any misgivings; the course of my research just happened to switch more directly into the human sphere. However, when the time came, there was a feeling of relief at no longer being compelled to do dog research. I always had a feeling of some guilt at the conclusion of each experiment as I injected a lethal dose of barbiturate into the animal. You see, I come from a family of dog lovers.

This is not to imply that my forebears rode to hounds or that we were all "good ole boys" who bravely went out into the forest with their dogs to shoot deer, bear, or occasionally one another. On the contrary, I came from a long line of city dwellers, and the nearest forebear to me, my father, was neither heroic nor athletically inclined. His date of birth made him too young for World War I and too old for World War II, so there were no opportunities for military exploits. The one time he even mentioned military service to his sons was at the outbreak of World War II when he gave the routine speech about us taking care of mom should he have to go into the army. Our response, almost in unison, was one of immediate assurance. "Dad, they'll be taking women and children before they ever take you!"

As for athletics, the most strenuous sport my dad ever indulged in involved placing a penny on the crack between two sidewalk squares of concrete and bouncing a rubber ball back and forth between himself and his opponent, trying to rack up points by hitting the coin in the process.

My dad did surprise us some years before, however, when our first dog, Teddy, inspired him to perform the only notable heroic *and* athletic act we can recall. In fact, this act redeemed him in our uncompromising children's eyes for all the years to come despite his forlorn physique and our irrepressible desire to kid him about it when the opportunity arose.

Teddy, a black and white spitz, was found wandering on the streets of New York and assumed to be an unwanted stray. Actually he had been lost by his owner who continued to search for his whereabouts weeks after we had picked him up at the pound and adopted him.

I do not recall if the original owner ever made a formal request for return of the dog and been refused. What I do vividly recall is a particular summer evening when my father, older brother, and I took Teddy for a walk. I was relaxed and held Teddy loosely on the leash. Suddenly a car pulled up beside the curb. A man jumped out of the front passenger's seat, yanked the leash out of my hand, lifted Teddy into his arms, and jumped back into the car.

Before the car and its contents could disappear into the night, my father rushed forward and leaped onto the running board—they still had them in those days—commandeering the vehicle to a halt. A policeman was called to the scene of the attempted dognapping.

It later turned out that the man who snatched Teddy was truly his legal owner and could prove it. We lost the dog, but my father's fearless performance and our adulation of it were the rewards of the episode. In following years other beloved dogs cheered my childhood, and later still others attached themselves to my own children after I grew into maturity, marriage, and fatherhood.

My experiences with dogs as experimental subjects began in 1961, near the start of my two-year fellowship in cardiovascular research at the University of Utah School of Medicine in Salt Lake City, Utah. As a medical resident, I had become interested in polycythemia and the potential adverse hemodynamic effects of this excessive production of red blood cells. Cardiac catheterization of polycythemic patients was not ordinarily considered justifiable, so I and another trainee decided to utilize dogs before and after artificial polycythemia, induced by red cell transfusions. My coinvestigator and I were cognizant of the effects that anesthesia might have on our results, so we decided to include some awake dogs as part of the study in addition to those anesthetized throughout the procedure. Furthermore, we were keen to determine the effects of exercise upon the circulatory effects of polycythemia. To accomplish this, we recognized that we would have to train some dogs to run on a treadmill while we attempted to measure pressures and flows utilizing indwelling catheters, placed under anesthesia some days before.

It was not an easy task we had set for ourselves. We still had to see patients in hospital, do consultations, attend clinics, assist with human catheterizations in patients, read electrocardiograms for two hospitals, and perform all the other duties required of us as part of our training in cardiology. But youthful energy, inexperience, and ambition can be great spurs to physical effort. With each new shipment of new dogs to the animal care facility of the medical school, we attempted to sort out the most likely candidates for the conscious, exercising component of the project. We needed dogs that were sturdy, friendly, and most important, capable of learning how to run the treadmill for us.

Eventually four dogs were selected, and each evening, after our hospital chores had been completed, we could be found on the hospital grounds running with the dogs to keep them in good physical shape. After they had warmed up a bit on the hospital lawn, the dogs were taken into the laboratory for attempts at treadmill training. I do not remember much about the first two dogs we used because the training period had clearly not been long enough. They barely managed to stay on the treadmill with the data obtained usable but not ideal. To insure more optimal results in the second pair, we subjected them to a much longer preparatory period and as a result inevitably became attached to them.

The first was a husky but totally nondescript mélange of breeds who richly deserved the nickname we gave him, Mutt. The other was a magnificent German shepherd, nearly colt sized who, despite his great mass and ferocious appearance was completely docile, friendly, and even a little goofy. We named him Jeff after the other member of the old comic strip duo. Both dogs performed splendidly for us throughout the experiment. At the conclusion of each segment, however, we only administered enough anesthetic to enable us to remove the catheters without causing any discomfort and sewing up the wounds under sterile conditions.

We finally worked up enough courage to go see the chief of medicine and ask him if we could not simply take these two wonderful dogs, to whom we owed so much, up into the surrounding hills and release them in the hopes that someone might adopt them. The request was refused. The law, written or not, was that experimental animals, once having served this purpose, had to be sacrificed. Not being able to perform the act myself, I had one of the animal handlers do the deed some days later.

As fate would have it, my subsequent dog studies were all performed under general anesthesia. These all involved advancing cardiac catheters to very specific sites within the coronary circulation, delicate operations that never could be accomplished were the dogs awake. In these experiments, all acute and performed in unconscious animals, there was no chance of establishing the kind of bonds that had been forged with Mutt and Jeff.

One might ask why we singled out dogs for this type of work and unusually large ones? The answer is that mice, rats, cats, and even small dogs had vessels too small for the insertion of the catheters we used for hemodynamic measurements. In some respects the coronary circulation of pigs is closer to that of man than that of dogs, and on one or two occasions, I assisted other investigators in performing such studies. But pigs tend to be a little unwieldy in the laboratory and much more expensive than our mongrel dogs were.

In one study, in order to evaluate how comparable our experimental results in dogs might be to humans, we chose to study large male baboons. Not only were the prices for these animals truly exorbitant, but their vessels tended to go into spasm as one handled them, making catheter insertions quite difficult. Finally, they seemed to sense what was in store for them, and I had to assist the "dieners" in restraining them as we administered the intravenous anesthetic. Luckily the bites and scratches we sustained did not result in some horrible disease later overtaking us.

So it was large mongrel dogs who constituted my experimental population over the years. While I maintained a distaste for dispatching them as I did at the end, I was at least somewhat comforted by the knowledge that had we not purchased these dogs and ended their lives with intravenous barbiturates, they would have met a far more horrible end at many of the dog pounds where death by asphyxiation in so-called "decompression chambers" awaited them. (Fortunately this practice, to my knowledge, is generally outlawed at present.)

Animal rights activists have violently protested against "mindless" experimentation on defenseless creatures. But as I look back over the decades I spent in the animal laboratory, I remain convinced that there could have been no substitutes for the dogs I have sacrificed to research. Beyond the modest contributions of our own cardiovascular research, one can point to major advances in the treatment of coronary heart disease, pacemaking, cardiac resuscitation, and transplantation, to mention but a few, that would never have been accomplished without the use of dogs. They and other experimental animals have all provided vital knowledge, not only to those interested in cardiovascular research, but endocrinology, pharmaceuticals, infectious disease, and just about every other aspect of human biology.

This is not to deny that there have been animal abuses in medical research. In response to these, and in all candor probably the antivivisectionist onslaught as well, scientific organizations and government agencies have set up stringent standards for the humane treatment of animals used for experimental purposes and instituted effective means of monitoring compliance with them.

One must not forget, however, that the ultimate experimental animal is man himself. Ironically, it is often those who spend much of their lives in animal experimentation who turn up, along with family members, as the first human volunteers when this Rubicon of research must ultimately be crossed. (Some of the more memorable accounts of human auto-experimentation may be found in Lawrence K. Altman's well-researched book, *Who Goes First?*)

Therefore, when someone utters "mindless" in regard to animal research, I am not reminded of those engaged in this important work. It is not them we should rail against. It is the intellectual bigots who throughout history have prevented innovation and punished independent thought. It is the book burners and the people burners that constitute the threat to us all. These and the perverted fanatics who break into laboratories and destroy the fruits of years of painstaking investigation and analysis.

And yet, despite my unwavering support for animal research, there remains a residue of remorse over the way I have disposed of so many dogs, these engaging and trusting animals of which I have always been inordinately fond. I read somewhere that, at least in the past, the students and medical faculty in Osaka, Japan, made an annual pilgrimage to honor the experimental animals they had sacrificed in the preceding year. Perhaps these lines I have written is a form of personal expiation, my own way of paying my respects to Mutt and Jeff and all the other fine dogs who have contributed so much to scientific knowledge and the betterment of humankind.

11

"Non-Cognitive" Comes Home to Roost

> cognitive: adj. pertaining to the mental processes of perception, memory, judgement and reasoning.
> —*Random House Dictionary of the English Language,* 2nd ed.

THE FIRST TIME I heard about non-cognitive physicians was a few years back at a monthly meeting of our Department of Medicine. Since then the term has cropped up increasingly in the medical literature or at meetings—especially those attended by nonsurgeons.

Mention of the term is usually accompanied by a smug smile and acknowledged with similar smirks and head nodding of all those nonsurgeons in the audience who, unquestionably, have long harbored a resentment toward our surgical colleagues. To some extent such an attitude may be justified. After all, surgeons are no more worthy than the rest of us even though they achieve more public recognition and significantly more money, no small thing in a money-oriented society where earning power, more than anything else, determines how high or low one fits into the social scale.

I must admit to being a frequent nodder along with my fellow internists, although my smile at poking fun has perhaps not been quite so wide or malicious as those around me. After all, I owe my life to a surgeon. As a medical student, I was surgically cured of a malignant tumor after months of visits to reputable internists failed to convince them that I was harboring this threat to my life. Professional jealousy tends to diminish considerably in the wake of such a devastating personal experience.

As a student I even toyed with the idea of becoming a surgeon. Their aggressive approach to disease I often found much more to my liking than the fiddle-faddling characteristic of some internists. The ones I trained under often seemed preoccupied, observing their patients with morbid fascination and making copious notes while the patients simply "went down the tubes."

Ultimately, I decided against a surgical career. I felt that I just did not have the feet for it; my susceptible arches simply could not bear the weight of two or three hours at a clip in the operating room. (The fact that, as an academic cardiologist, I later found myself spending five or six hours doing a study in the cardiac catheterization laboratory—and with a ten pound lead apron on to boot—is one of life's ironies over which I continue to chuckle.)

Yet, throughout my private life, I have frequently been reminded about what it means *not* to be a surgeon. At nonmedical social functions when I identify myself as a cardiologist, the response of many lay persons is, "Oh, so you operate on hearts?" My reply in the negative, despite a sincere effort to convince them that my efforts on the patients' behalf really are of some importance, invariably results in the evaporation of that incipient glow of admiration and respect that I had initially detected in my opposite.

How could it be otherwise? When was the last time you read a novel or saw a film about doctors who were *not* surgeons? Fictional work always concerns some surgeon who undergoes a crisis in his life—it is always a "he"—before emerging at the conclusion even more brilliant and admirable than ever. Perhaps it is a great surgeon losing a dear patient through only one isolated error in an otherwise spotless career. Or perhaps it concerns one of his acolytes developing some new operation for the conquest of a previously incurable condition. These are infinitely more gripping than one about a dermatologist who mistakes poison ivy for poison oak or finds he has been treating a patient for atopic dermatitis when it really was psoriasis. And, by the way, can you recall a single nonsurgeon who ever appeared regularly in a major role on the television hit, *MASH?*

While the rest of us in medicine have remained either vaguely or explicitly resentful of all this undeserved adulation, the surgeons, for their part, have remained, at least outwardly, pretty tolerant of us "medical creeps." After all, they say that living well is the best revenge, and surgeons are surely very much aware that it might not be too wise to offend those upon whom they depend for referrals.

Suggesting that surgeons, just because they visibly *do things* to patients more than the rest of us, are nonthinking, harks back to medieval times when medical savants theorized about airs and vapors, continued to read from Galen, and remained perched in high chairs directing dissection down below without even approaching the objects of their anatomy students' concern.

Meanwhile barber-surgeons, considered unworthy of any academic respect, attended more directly to the needs of many patients. Of course they bungled oftentimes, just as the medical doctors did, but they also included the likes of Ambroise Paré. And in later years, surgeons such as John Hunter obviously contributed a great deal more to our understanding and treatment of disease than many of their medical contemporaries.

My own epiphany about the injustice of such attitudes of internists toward surgeons arose from an article in which the considerable financial return of a "procedure-oriented" medical subspecialty, gastroenterology, was contrasted with that of a "cognitive-oriented" medical subspecialty, rheumatology.[1] The conclusion of the study was that, considered as a financial decision, training in rheumatology and other "cognitive-oriented" medical specialties was a "poor investment."

What these authors were saying about gastroenterology could certainly be applied to cardiologists, and, as one of the latter, I was acutely aware of being tarred with the same irresponsible brush that had been applied to the surgeons. I now saw clearly the injustice of implying that the act of opening up our patients' bodies or peering within their cavities with the assistance of endoscopic devices in order to diagnose or treat them was essentially not preceded, accompanied, or followed by any meaningful thought processes. Of course, such assumptions are as insulting as they are untrue. I must add that I am also offended by surgical apologists who suggest that their higher incomes are simply the result of working longer or harder.[2]

In my own field, it is a lot easier to schedule our patients' coronary bypass operations than the onset of their coronary occlusions. It is true that the schedules of trauma surgeons, obstetricians, orthopedists, and many general surgeons are often at the mercy of chance catastrophes, but the professional lives of eye surgeons, plastic surgeons, and others within the specialty are infinitely better regulated than those of busy internists, pediatricians, and family practitioners.

There is no doubt that financial rewards are skewed toward those whose practices are procedure oriented, and it is only proper that some attempt be made at addressing this imbalance. The Resource-Based Relative Value Scale (RBRVS) was certainly a step in this direction, and provided we can all bone up sufficiently on advanced mathematics to understand it and install main frame computers in our offices to implement it, perhaps it will accomplish its purpose. Beyond all this, the recently reported multimillion-dollar incomes and bonuses of HMO executives is a much more egregious example of maldistribution of medical profits, but that is another story.

In the meantime, by continually bickering about income, we run the risk of appearing to the observant public to be in the same league as that genre of medical carpetbaggers, not to mention the executives of many American corporations who run their companies into the ground, exit with the rewards of "golden parachute" deals, and continue to complain about unfair competition from Japan where more effective executives receive only a fraction of that awarded to their American counterparts.

The standard reply to the complaining nonsurgeon has been "if he wanted a surgeon's income, he should have become a surgeon in the first place." Thank goodness, the financial "penalty" of not becoming a surgeon is not all that severe, and physicians continue to do much better than the vast majority of other Americans in economic terms. Furthermore, preoccupation with personal income deflects from grappling with much larger problems with the health care system in this country.

The last time I checked, physicians' income accounted for only about 20 percent of the national health cost. Reducing their income by as much as a third would reduce the total cost of medical care by only about 7 percent, hardly a dent in the overall problem. Rather than our own incomes, we should be concerned about our inability to control the costs of the medical economic tiger of which we are, apparently, only the tail. We should concentrate on doing this without having to reduce the quality of care to those patients who are insured; we should also find ways to make adequate and affordable care available to those who cannot afford it, over 37 million strong and growing.

Historically, the American medical profession has seemed inordinately prone and incredibly adept at shooting itself in the collective foot. The plea here is to let the wounds heal and direct our combined efforts to more appropriate goals in solving our nation's health care problems in the future.

Notes

1. Prashker MJ and Meenan RF. Subspecialty training: Is it financially worthwhile? Annals Int Med 1991; 115:715–719.
2. Maloney JV Jr. A critical analysis of the resource-based relative value scale. JAMA 1991; 226:3453–3458.

12

Bats in the Belfry or Bugs in the Belly?

Helicobacter and the Resurrection of Johannes Fibiger

THIS IS A story about two men, three diseases, and what we may have learned from them over the past one hundred years. The men are Johannes Fibiger (1867–1928), a pathologist in Copenhagen, and Barry J. Marshall (1951–), an internist-gastroenterologist from Australia. The diseases are peptic ulcer, gastritis, and gastric cancer.

Let us begin with the career of Johannes Andreas Grib Fibiger, the Danish pathologist who was working at the University of Copenhagen at the beginning of this century. In 1907 he discovered stomach tumors in three wild rats. On sectioning these papillomatous growths, he discovered within them the presence of worms (nematodes) of the *gongylonema* type he later reclassified as *Spiroptera neoplastica*. Searching earlier literature about them, he learned that part of their life cycle included ingestion by cockroaches. He surmised that the rats he had dissected had become infected with the nematode by eating a particular species of cockroach that had carried the larval form of the worm. Thus the cockroach had served as an intermediary host before being consumed by the rats with maturing of the worm in their stomachs and the eventual result of tumor formation.

His initial attempts at discovering other rats with these tumors were disheartening—over a thousand were trapped and autopsied with no success. Finally, in a rat-infested sugar refinery in Copenhagen, forty of sixty rats trapped had nematode infestation, and among these, seven had demonstrated growths within the stomach that Fibiger interpreted as cancer. Roaches trapped in the same refinery were found to contain the larval stage of the worm. By feeding such infected cockroaches to rats, he was able to produce stomach tumors in about 20 percent of them. He later uncovered what he believed to be lung metastases spreading from the stomach cancers. By 1913 he was able to publish his results, first with a brief report in German,[1] and then in greater detail in Danish,[2] and then in French[3] as well. His experimental model of stomach cancer had important implications about the genesis of human malignancy for all who cared to read between the lines, although Fibiger never was too explicit in his remarks regarding this.

However, at a time when cancer was already recognized as a major cause of human illness and mortality, and when cancer research up to that time was not too productive, Fibiger's findings were looked upon as a major breakthrough in understanding the pathogenesis of this dreaded disease. It is easy to discount such a connection on the eve of the twenty-first century, but at the beginning of the twentieth, when most human populations were much more widely affected by worm infestation, such a connection did not seem farfetched in the least. After all, in 1911, A. R. Ferguson had reported an association between urinary bladder infection with schistosomes (bilharziasis) and the subsequent development of bladder cancer among Egyptian men,[4] a finding which has been found to hold true even today. Could Fibiger's findings not represent another link between infection and cancer?

In the 1919 edition of the influential Ewing textbook on neoplastic disease,[5] Fibiger's work was termed a "brilliant study." Admiration for this research seemed universal and finally led the Nobel Committee to award Fibiger the prize for Physiology and Medicine in 1926. At the ceremony the presenter could not have been more effusive in his praise, describing Fibiger's work as "immortal," and quoting another expert in cancer research who referred to it as "the greatest contribution to experimental medicine in our generation."[6]

Not all within the medical research community were so convinced. Indeed, early on, contemporaries of Fibiger pointed out that the injection of chemical or mechanical irritants into the stomachs of rats could produce lesions similar to those described by Fibiger.[7] It was also pointed out that the tumors described by Fibiger had not been shown to have the true characteristics of cancers, continuing to grow following the removal of the supposed initially inciting factor. The need for control groups as part of such investigations was not generally appreciated at the time, and therefore Fibiger did not include a group of rats of the same species, housed and fed and treated identically in every way except for worm infestation, to compare with his infected group.

The diet fed the rats was especially suspect, and finally, in 1936, Passey and his collaborators at the University of Leeds demonstrated that by feeding a diet similar to that used by Fibiger, and found to be deficient in vitamin A, lung lesions identical to those described by Fibiger could be produced.[8] Other disturbing reports appeared prompting the 1940 edition of Ewing to express "serious doubt on the validity of Fibiger's interpretations."[9] Perhaps the coup de grâce was delivered in 1952 when investigators at the University of Minnesota closely duplicated Fibiger's protocol with the addition of two control groups: one without worm infestation also fed the vitamin deficient diet and one with worm infestation but provided a fully nutritious diet.[10] Although the most marked changes appeared in the infected rats with the vitamin deficient diet, the vitamin deficient rats without worms were also found to develop stomach lesions. The worm infected rats with a nutritious diet had only minimal stomach changes. None of the stomach lesions produced seemed to meet the histological criteria of carcinoma, and whatever changes that were induced in the stomach were more closely related to dietary deficiency than worm infestation.

The impact of all this on subsequent Nobel committees can only be surmised. Suffice it to note that it was forty years before another Nobel Prize for Medicine and Physiology was awarded for achievements in cancer research. This was in 1966 when Charles Huggins received the award for his introduction of the hormonal treatment of prostate cancer. Huggins shared the prize with Peyton Rous of the Rockefeller Institute who in 1911 had reported the transfer of chicken sarcomas with a cell-free filtrate[11] and whose work, ironically, had been gently but summarily dismissed by Fibiger in his own Nobel address.[12] Rous was eighty-seven when his early demonstration of the potential for viral induction of cancer was finally officially honored; he had been considered and rejected for the award over twenty times during the preceding four decades.

With the passage of time, Fibiger's story has tended to be forgotten. Whenever plucked out of the past by some medical historian or commentator, it has often been looked upon with some embarrassment, irony, and, at times, even bemusement. However, given Fibiger's commitment to science, his honesty and extraordinary industry on its behalf, a sense of tragedy should also be added. His memory demands it—and perhaps a little bit more, given more recent developments in our understanding of the links between infection and cancer.

Let us now shift the scene to Australia and the Royal Perth Hospital in the latter part of 1980. Barry Marshall, twenty-nine-year-old medical registrar (the equivalent of our hospital internal medicine fellows), was about to begin a six-month elective on the gastrointestinal service as part of his training program in internal medicine. Research was required as part of the training, and he inquired about the possibilities of engaging in such work.[13]

An initial suggestion to do an analysis of the clinical work of the GI section did not seem promising. However, a second opportunity was presented in the form of a page torn from an ordinary lined notepad. On it were listed the names of about twenty patients whose stomach biopsies had been examined by the hospital pathologist, Dr. J. Robin Warren. All had had, in association with diagnostic endoscopy, small biopsies obtained from their stomachs for a variety of complaints, most often the presence of an ulcer or inflammation (gastritis).

The main purpose of obtaining these tissue samples was to distinguish ordinary peptic ulcer, gastritis, or benign growths from possible stomach cancer masquerading as such. But it was something quite different that had caught Warren's attention. It was the presence of spiral-shaped organisms that he had found nestling on the surface of the stomach lining (epithelium) just beneath the mucous layer that protected it from the acidic stomach contents. It also turned out that these organisms produced urease, which could convert urea in the surrounding area to the alkaline ammonium hydroxide, providing additional protection. These were not easy to detect with the standard hematoxylin and eosin stains ordinarily utilized for this purpose, but Warren found that silver staining techniques easily revealed them in abundance in many of the patients whose specimens had been sent to him for examination. What were these organisms doing there? What specific type of microorganism did they represent? Were they initiators of pathology or only "innocent onlookers" after the fact. What Warren needed was a clinician to make the proper correlations with the clinical stories of these patients, and Marshall would prove to be that person.

There had been scattered reports of "spirochetal" organisms found in stomachs subjected to autopsy examination previously, some dating back fifty years or more. However, by the mid-fifties, these had been essentially discounted as contaminants or opportunistic organisms that had populated the stomach after disease had set in and were unrelated to the underlying pathologic processes present. The introduction of upper gastrointestinal endoscopy in the sixties and seventies to allow direct visualization of stomach pathology during life, and then the acquisition of small biopsies by forceps attachments to these instruments indirectly opened this whole question once again. Warren, according to his junior collaborator, was just the kind of person to seize upon this opportunity. Warren's meticulous examination of the specimens sent to him would provide the opening wedge for some rather remarkable new developments in the field of gastroenterology.

Before Warren and Marshall could embark on a highly structured prospective study of the problem, a number of preliminary preparations were necessary. As a result of these, the ability to stain fresh mucosal specimens with ordinary Gram stains to reveal the organisms was one important finding. After researching the literature and reexamining the specimens obtained, the coinvestigators felt that what they were seeing under the microscope were really organisms of the *Campylobacter* type, and a previous report on methodology for culturing them was adopted. (In 1989, on the basis of further investigations, it was found that the stomach bacteria with which they had been dealing were distinct from the Campylobacter genus. *Helicobacter pylori* was the new designation given to these organisms[14] and will be used in reference to them throughout the remainder of this review.)

By the beginning of 1982, they undertook what they planned to be the study of one hundred consecutive patients undergoing gastroscopy for a number of clinical complaints. The beauty of the plan, according to Marshall, was that now, for the first time, specimens could be obtained from "normal" patients, those with symptoms found to be unrelated to a specific stomach pathology, and their results in terms of *H. pylori* infection could be compared to patients whose symptoms had been connected to a specific cause. In the course of the study, Warren would be blinded to the clinical histories of the patients whose specimens he would be examining. Statistical analysis would be provided by appropriate university collaborators to ensure the reliability of their data.

For the microbiological analytic portion of the study, Marshall recalls that he was not exactly received in the laboratory with unbounded enthusiasm. His project was relegated to the "fecal lab" in a corner of the facility, and there were frequent changes in the assignment of laboratory technicians to his project, making the development of their proper orientation in the project and the reliability in their results difficult to achieve.

The initiation of the laboratory study was depressing. Time and again Marshall would see organisms on Gram staining the fresh specimens, but nothing positive was ever reported culture positive from the laboratory. The breakthrough was finally achieved through a series of events—surprisingly unrecognized by Marshall—highly reminiscent of Alexander Fleming's discovery of the effects of *Penicillium* mold on bacterial growth in a nearly discarded culture plate after a holiday interlude over fifty years earlier in 1928.

Culture of stomach material was not an ordinary function of the bacteriology laboratory. Most often the specimens obtained had been for the purpose of establishing the presence of the more ordinary types of infections that periodically plague hospitals and the communities they serve, outbreaks of staphylococcal disease and the like. It turns out that the material obtained from Marshall was being treated in a manner similar to that obtained from throat swabs in upper respiratory infections. Among these, it was well known that if no pathogen had grown out by the second or third day, the culture plates would soon be covered with overgrowth by any number of commensal organisms known to be present in the normal oropharynx. The plates would be useless diagnostically. Therefore if no positive results were uncovered by the second or third day, the plates would be discarded. Unrecognized by Marshall, his plates were being thrown out by the laboratory technicians after thirty-six to forty-eight hours, even though, as is usually the case with gastric specimens, they were still quite clean. Unrecognized by the laboratory technicians was the fact that the organisms he was hoping to culture might be relatively slow growing, requiring four or five days before becoming evident upon the culture plates.

A four-day extended weekend Easter holiday proved providential. The harried technician assigned to quickly examine all the results from the previous Thursday and Friday skipped over Marshall's specimens that Saturday morning in order to pay proper attention to more pressing clinical problems. Following the holiday, when the full staff appeared for duty and the culture of Marshall's thirty-seventh patient was examined properly, there the H. pylori colonies had blossomed forth, pristine and uncontaminated. No overgrowth had appeared because in the process of performing the endoscopy, the acid contents of the stomach had essentially sterilized the tubing, eliminating any other possible organisms that may have contaminated it during insertion. Only the acid-resistant H. pylori were able to survive.

As the results of their work began to be tabulated, the implication of H. pylori in gastric pathology began to become quite clear to Marshall and Warren. They recognized the importance of establishing their priority in uncovering this radically new connection in the field of gastroenterology and in 1983 contacted the widely disseminated British Journal, Lancet, to give notice of their line of investigation in the letters to editor section. In the June 4, 1983, issue, there were actually two letters submitted under the title "Unidentified Curved Bacilli on Gastric Epithelium in Active Chronic Gastritis."[15] The first letter, by Warren, described the pathological findings and was limited to statements emphasizing the fact that bacteria could exist within the stomach of such patients, contrary to previous beliefs about the sterility of that organ. In a second letter, Marshall, ten years or more younger than his conservative collaborator in pathology, was much less restrained in his comments about the implications of their findings. His final sentence, in essence, threw down the gauntlet at the feet of much of what had become established dogma in the field of gastroenterology: "If these bacteria are truly associated with antral gastritis, as described by Warren, they may have a part to play in other poorly understood, gastritis disease (i.e., peptic ulcer and gastric cancer)." Note the final word.

Although it was gastritis that had initially drawn Warren's attention to his pathological findings in the stomach, it was peptic ulcer, especially that occurring in the duodenum, that had impressed Marshall. It was duodenal ulcer, after all, rather than those occurring in the stomach, that accounted for the overwhelming number of ulcers with which clinicians had to deal. Later that year, at an infectious disease meeting in Brussels, Marshall made his first major presentation outside of Australia about their findings with H. pylori, and especially the implications this had in the way physicians generally looked upon peptic ulcer disease. In June of 1984, the results of Marshall and Warren's work on their first hundred patients appeared in Lancet and clearly demonstrated the strong link between H. pylori infection and gastritis, gastric ulcers, and duodenal ulcers.[16]

The possibility of any bacteria infecting the stomach, no less a role for them in the genesis of peptic ulcers, simply refuted all that medical people had been brought up to believe about normal and abnormal gastric physiology. It all harked back to Col. William Beaumont, a U.S. Army surgeon, and his studies involving Alexis St. Martin, a patient afflicted with a gastric fistula to the abdominal wall, courtesy of an unfortunate gun shot accident. Beaumont had not been the first or last investigator to study such fistulae, but he had been the most persistent and systematic. He included his findings in a book entitled *Experiments and Observations on the Gastric Juice and the Physiology of Di-*

gestion, published in 1833. In it he established basic concepts about gastric juice and digestion that have persisted up to the present and been embellished on by an entire school of gastrointestinal physiologists, clinicians, and even psychiatrists.

Importantly, he established clearly for the first time that the stomach contents were indeed acidic. With the help of cooperating chemists, analysis of the stomach fluid obtained from St. Martin showed the presence of muriatic (hydrochloric) acid. Combined with gastric peristalsis ("a constant disturbance, or *churning* of the contents"), according to Beaumont, this characterized the gastric environment as one wherein "even the hardest bone cannot withstand its action." He was also explicit about the effects of emotion on the stomach: "In febrile diathesis or predisposition from whatever cause . . . fear, anger or whatever depresses or disturbs the nervous system, the villous coat becomes sometimes red and dry, at other times pale and moist, and loses its smooth healthy appearance."[17]

Such concepts introduced by Beaumont and carried on by his successors convinced all students of medicine, even up to the present, that the stomach was, in a way, a wonder of nature, a seething caldron contained within us that miraculously was prevented from digesting its host and governed by a psyche that might one day run amuck and lead to peptic ulceration and other dire malfunctions.

Although it was well realized that some intruders such as *salmonella* or the cholera vibrio might manage to survive the perilous passage in order to work their mischief further down along the gastrointestinal tract, it was impossible to conceive of any organism actually capable of "setting up housekeeping" in such a hostile territory. Yet this is precisely what Warren and Marshall were proving to be the case. This was neatly managed by the bacteria sequestering themselves between the endothelial lining of the stomach and the protective mucous coat that provided a barrier between them and the gastric contents. Furthermore, H. pylori turns out to be a urease-producing organism. It can break down urea in the environment ultimately to form the alkaline ammonium hydroxide, a further protection against excessive acid contact.

As for proof of the role of H. pylori in the causation of peptic ulcer, a detailed recounting is beyond the scope of this essay. Suffice it to say that it was ultimately shown that the association between *Helicobacter* peptic ulceration was, with few exceptions explained by other circumstances (e.g., nonsteroidal anti-inflammatory drug administration), invariable. Furthermore, treatment of peptic ulcers with appropriate antibiotics aimed against this organism resulted in excellent responses with relapses rare while conventional treatment of peptic ulcer with antacids and drugs to reduce acid secretion often resulted in recurrence. Ironically, some of the studies showing this difference in effectiveness were carried out by the most vocal and influential of Marshall's early critics.[18]

There was, however, one aspect of all this work that continued to trouble Marshall. Time and again, from the very beginning, he would be asked the traditional chicken-and-egg question: how could he be sure that H. pylori, seen in all these cases of gastritis and peptic ulcer, actually *preceded* the gastritis and peptic ulcers? Could it be that the H. pylori infected the stomach only after the pathological environment made the stomach more receptive to them? Marshall attempted to create a number of animal models to demonstrate the causative role of the organism, but all of these proved impractical, cumbersome, or unconvincing. He finally fell back on the one animal he could fully rely upon, himself.

After undergoing gastroscopy and having his own gastric mucosa sampled to prove he was normal, he obtained H. pylori from the stomach of a patient with chronic gastritis. After successfully culturing the organism, he gathered up the colonies in a bacteriological draft and downed it. A week later, symptoms began to appear, and following a repeat biopsy of his stomach, the lining was shown to be inflamed and densely populated with the organisms. Thanks to a sturdy constitution and perhaps the antibiotics his wife insisted he take later on, Marshall survived the episode without sequelae and has remained in good health ever since. As a result of this self-experimentation, he had fulfilled all of Koch's postulates related to proof of an etiologic infectious agent: he had obtained it from an affected individual, isolated it in culture, transferred it to a second individual, and produced the same pathology as a result. A description of this episode appeared in The Medical Journal of Australia in April 1985[19] along with an expanded report of the demonstrated association of H. pylori with gastrointestinal disease among 267 patients, normal and abnormal, who had undergone evaluation by Marshall and his colleagues.[20]

We now turn to Marshall's suggestion about the association between H. pylori infection and stomach cancer. If his views on peptic ulcer had been initially received as seditious to the defenders of traditional gastrointestinal dogma, his suggestions regarding cancer must have seemed downright subversive, especially in view of the whole Fibiger debacle.

Again there was the problem of the chicken or the egg, but this time the solution was provided by investigators other than Marshall. It turns out that in the mid-sixties, the Kaiser Health Plan in California had collected and frozen the sera of over 120,000 of its subscribers. When, over the next few decades, 109 of these individuals developed adenocarcinoma of the stomach, 84 percent were shown by serological testing of their blood samples, obtained years before the tumors, to have been H. pylori positive.[21] A similar study performed among Japanese American men in Hawaii showed the same sort of results,[22] and both studies appeared in the *New England Journal of Medicine* in 1991. An editorial accompanying these major reports was entitled "Is Gastric Carcinoma an Infectious Disease?"[23]

Although many patients in the control populations in California and Hawaii also harbored the bacteria in their stomachs and did not develop gastric cancer, one would have to agree with the editorialist that other factors are probably involved. Nonetheless H. pylori was established in both places as a major player, and in 1993, the Eurogast Study, an epidemiological analysis of seventeen different countries, reported approximately a six-fold increased risk of gastric cancer among populations with 100 percent H. pylori infection.[24] Finally, it should be noted that, although gastric cancer is a rare cancer in the continental United States where Helicobacter infection is uncommon, worldwide, cancer of the stomach in repeated cancer surveys is the first or second most commonly occurring malignancy.[25]

In addition to stomach cancer, H. pylori has been found in association with a low-grade stomach tumor, a mucous-associated lymphoid tissue (MALT) lymphoma.[26] Treatment of these tumors with antibiotics aimed at H. pylori has resulted in marked regression of these tumors. It is too early to tell whether or not cures will ultimately be obtained by such treatment.

Where does all this place Fibiger in the context of what we now know about infection and cancer? In a review about the association between parasites and cancer published in 1963,[27] and now considered something of a classic on the subject, W. S. Bailey pointed out that as far back as 1906, it was shown that another worm, *Taenia taeniaformis*, was known to cause liver cancer in the rat. Bailey also noted that in 1955, it was discovered that a close cousin of Fibiger's nematode, *Spirocerca lupi*, could cause the development of sarcomas following esophageal infestation in dogs.

When one surveys the entire spectrum of infection and human cancer at present (Table 12.1), aside from gastric carcinoma, there is ample evidence for

Table 12.1 Infection and Other Human Neoplasia

Schistosomiasis	Bladder cancer
Hepatitis B	Hepatoma
Epstein-Barr Virus	Nasopharyngeal carcinoma
Papilloma virus	Cervical cancer
HIV	Kaposi's sarcoma, lymphoma
H. pylori	MALT lymphoma

the role of infective agents—albeit no nematodes—in the etiology of such diseases. How do they bring this about? It certainly seems clear that chronic infection may result in chronic inflammation such as occurs with chronic gastritis and stomach cancer with *Helicobacter*. Bladder cancer may occur in a similar way after *Schistosome* infection, while in other infection-associated neoplasms, such a connection does not seem operative, and other mechanisms must be involved. The role of infection in neoplasia is undeniable, and perhaps further associations will be made in the future, now that the concept is well established.

Given all this and Fibiger's long and distinguished service in other areas of pathology, one cannot argue with the remark a parasitologist friend made to me that, regarding *Spiroptera* carcinoma, "Fibiger may have been barking up the wrong tree, but he was still a Great Dane."

In reviewing the rise and fall of Fibiger's reputation and in view of subsequent scientific findings about the association between infection and cancer, the final comments of Paul D. Stolley and Tamar Lasky, in an article they recently wrote concerning Fibiger, seem most fitting: "Today his story serves to remind us of the many blind alleys down which science must wander in the search for truth. It also illustrates the ease with which intelligent and educated scientists can mistake illusion for truth. With hindsight, we can spot the blind alleys of yesteryear, but who can say which are the blind alleys of today?"[28]

Notes

1. Fibiger J. Über eine durch Nematoden (Spiroptera sp.n.) hervorgerufene papillomatöse und karzinomatose Geschwulstbildung im Magen der Ratte. Berliner Tierarztliche Wochenschrift 1913; 20:368.

2. Fibiger J. Undersøgelser over en Nematode (Spiroptera sp.n.) og dens Evne til at fremkalde papillomatøse og carcinomatøse Svulster i Rottens Ventrikel. Hospitalstidende 1913; 6 (16):417–431.

3. Fibiger J. Recherches sur un nematode et sur sa faculté de provoquer des néoformations papillomateuses et carcinomateuses dans l'estomac du rat. Acad Royale Sci Lettres Danemark 1913; 1–41.

4. Ferguson AR. Associated bilharziosis and primary malignant disease of the urinary bladder, with observations on a series of forty cases. J Path and Bact 1911; 16:76–94.

5. Ewing J. *Neoplastic Diseases: A Text-Book on Tumors*. Philadelphia, Pa.: W. B. Saunders, 1919, 133–134.

6. Wernstedt W. Presentation speech in Nobel Lectures: Physiology or Medicine. 1922–1941. Amsterdam: Elsevier, 1965: 119–121.

7. Bullock FD and Rhodenburg GL. Experimental "carcinomata" of animals and their relation to true malignant tumors. J Cancer Research 1918; 3:227–240.

8. Passey RD, Leese A, Knox JC. Bronchiectasis and metaplasia in the lung of the laboratory rat. J Path and Bact 1936; 42:425–434.

9. Ewing J. *Neoplastic Diseases: A Treatise on Tumors*, 4th ed. Philadelphia, Pa.: W. B. Saunders, 1940, 138.

10. Hitchcock CR and Bell ET. Studies on the nematode parasite, Gongylonema neoplasticum (Spiroptera neoplasticum) and avitminosis A in the forestomach of rats: comparison with Fibiger's results. J Natl Cancer Inst 1952; 12:1345–1387.

11. Rous P. A sarcoma of the fowl transmissible by an agent separable from the tumor cells. J Exp Med 1911; 13:397–411.

12. Fibiger J. Investigations on *Spiroptera* carcinoma and the experimental induction of cancer: Nobel Lecture, Dec. 12, 1927. In *Nobel Lectures: Physiology or Medicine, 1922–1941*. New York: Elsevier Publishing Co., 1965, 122–150.

13. Interview with Dr. Marshall in Bethesda, Md. on Feb. 14, 1996. Dr. Marshall also kindly reviewed this chapter prior to publication for accuracy regarding his own work.

14. Goodwin CS, Armstrong JA, Chilvers T et al. Transfer of *Campylobacter mustelae* to *Helicobacter* gen. nov. as *Helicobacter pylori* comb. nov. and *Helicobacter mustelae* comb nov. respectively. Intl J of Systematic Bacteriol 1989; 39:397–405.

15. Warren JR and Marshall BJ. Unidentified curved bacilli on gastric epithelium in active chronic gastritis. Lancet 1983; 1:1273–1275.

16. Marshall BJ and Warren JR. Unidentified curved bacilli in the stomach of patients with gastritis and peptic ulceration. Lancet 1984; 1:1311–1315.

17. Beaumont W. *Experiments and Observations on the Gastric Juice and the Physiology of Digestion*. Plattsburgh, N.Y.: F. P. Allen, 1833, 107.

18. Graham DY, Lew GM, Klein PD et al. Effect of treatment of *Helicobacter pylori* on the long-term recurrence of gastic or duodenal ulcer. A randomized, controlled study. Annals Int Med 1992; 116:705–708.

19. Marshall BJ, Armstrong JA, McGechnie DB, Glancy RJ. Attempt to fulfil Koch's postulates for pyloric campylobacter. Med J Aust 1985; 142:436–439.

20. Marshall BJ, McGechnie DB, Rogers PA, Glancy RJ. Pyloric campylobacter infection and gastroduodenal disease. Med J Aust 1985; 142:439–444.

21. Parsonnet J, Friedman GD, Vandersteen DP et al. *Helicobacter pylori* infection and the risk of gastric carcinoma. N Engl J Med 1991; 325:1127–1131.

22. Nomura A, Stemmerman GN, Chyou P et al. *Helicobacter pylori* infection and gastric carcinoma among Japanese Americans in Hawaii. N Engl J Med 1991; 325:1132–1136.

23. Correa P. Is gastric carcinoma an infectious disease? (Edit.) N Engl J Med 1991; 325:1170–1171.

24. The Eurogast Study Group. An international association between *Helicobacter pylori* infection and gastric cancer. Lancet 1993; 341:1359–1362.

25. Parkin DM, Laara E, Muir CS. Estimates of the worldwide frequency of sixteen major cancers in 1980. Intl J Cancer 1988; 41:184–187.

26. Wotherspoon AC, Ortiz-Hidalgo C, Falzon MR, Isaacson PG. *Helicobacter pylori* associated gastritis and primary B-cell gastric lymphoma. Lancet 1991; 338:1175–1176.

27. Bailey WS. Parasites and cancer. Annals NY Acad Sci 1963; 108:890–923.

28. Stolley PD and Lasky T. Johannes Fibiger and his Nobel prize for the hypothesis that a worm causes stomach cancer. Annals Int Med 1992; 116:765–769.

13

Whither Our Children?

I HAVE JUST returned from the bank where I have deposited one roll of dimes, one roll of nickels, and four rolls of pennies into a very special account. This represents a grand total of nine dollars, collected from the remains of pocket change over the last few months. It is not a lot of money by any standard, and it won't have any perceptible effect on our financial solvency. Notoriously careless with loose money about my person, I probably lose or misplace this much over the same course of time it took me to accumulate this amount. Yet, I still have the compulsion to remove the coins from my pockets each night and place them in an old cigarette box to await sorting, wrapping, and a trip to the bank. It gives me a great deal of pleasure, a sense of accomplishment.

The adult phase of my coin hoarding began over twenty years ago. I married fairly late in life, and while my two children were still toddlers, my contemporaries, who had married at much earlier ages, had children nearly in college. I soon began to hear the murmurs of anxiety mounting to wails of despair as these parents desperately began to search for the monetary wherewithal to fund their children's higher educations. Reports of canceled vacations, postponed new cars, and second mortgages became the lingua franca of my associates confronting the challenge of rising college costs.

Their complaints did not go unheeded by me. With only two children, ages two and four at the time, I thought I could head off such anxieties "at the bend" by a little simple financial planning early on. If only I put away my spare change each night, I reasoned, and periodically deposited the accumulated coinage to a special bank account for my kids, in the fifteen years or so it took to see them into kindergarten and out of high school, I would have accumulated enough, with added interest thrown in, to meet my future responsibilities successfully.

How naive could one be? I was like one of the characters in the musical, *The Pajama Game*, singing about that seven-and-a-half-cent raise ("Give it to me every hour, forty hours every week, and that's enough for me to be living like a king.") But at the end of one year of this Silas Marner kind of activity, with quarters thrown in as well at this stage, I found that only a little more than three hundred dollars had been saved.

These were the days when the cost of a year away at a name college was not yet in the neighborhood of twenty thousand dollars or more, but it could be foreseen that such a time was fast approaching. And then, of course, there would be the cost of their medical education, which we assumed would come next. With a prized but hardly utilitarian bachelor's degree in hand, my children would have to be supported through four years of medical school and possibly their residencies, in part, as well. Even as poor a mathematician as I could calculate a significant shortfall for my two children if I just kept on the same simplistic track of saving. My wife and I began peeling off substantial sums of our income and putting it away for the days when the kids would be college bound.

Our plans succeeded, at least the financial part to some degree. We haven't canceled a vacation; our cars are fairly current; our house is still our own. That is the good news. The downside is that neither of our two children will be going into medicine despite two physician parents deeply in love with their profession.

I am an academic cardiologist and my wife a radiologist in private practice. Neither of us would hesitate to do it all over again if the choice was to be made. We thought our enthusiasm would ignite a similar interest in our children. However, our daughter has chosen to become an English teacher (and a damned good one too), while our son started out by immersing himself for four years in economics. One year short of his master's degree in this discipline, he decided that he could not stand the prospect of spending the rest of his life looking at numbers; he determined that it was a veterinarian he wished to become. After two years of study to complete the required science courses he had originally abjured, he applied to and was accepted to veterinary school. As of this writing, he is in his third year at the University of Pennsylvania. Human and veterinary medicine not being all that different, we have lots in common to discuss upon his occasional returns to the fold on holiday, although it is not quite what I had in mind at the beginning.

Our own mistaken assumptions about what the career choices of our children might be raised considerations in my mind about the broad relationship between physicians in general and the professional aspirations of their children. Medicine bashing has become a favorite pastime of its practitioners for a litany of reasons you all know too well. Perhaps then it should come as no surprise that the children of today's physicians might not want to follow in their fathers' or mothers' footsteps.

In 1989, a telephone poll of one thousand physicians conducted by the Gallup people for the American Medical Association indicated that 25 percent of those contacted, knowing then what they did about the medicine of the present and the portents for the future, would probably not go to medical school if they had to do it all over again. Another 14 percent of those polled indicated that they *definitely* would not go into medicine again if they had to make the choice. With nearly 40 percent of practicing physicians giving off such negative signals, it would come as no surprise if the children of today's M.D.'s are turning to other pursuits or careers. Given the recent emergence of managed care, HMOs, and the like and their added negative effects upon physicians perceptions of the field, I suspect that a more recent poll might provide an even more negative response.

The problem that such data creates for me is that I have a hard time accepting it. We are a nation of world champion complainers; our ability to gripe—while getting the job done—might even be considered a national treasure. Thus, I felt a more meaningful reading of physicians' attitudes might be derived from the actions of their children either toward or away from the profession.

An irrepressible head counter, I decided to perform my own little survey a few years back, 1991 to be exact. If Gallup could poll a thousand physicians, then I certainly could handle 250, the number of full-time M.D.'s on our faculty at the New Jersey Medical School in Newark. To each was sent a questionnaire asking the following: how many children were in the family, the children's ages, and whether any of those college bound or beyond were either in medicine or aspiring to it. To detect any cultural differences, I separated the natural born Americans from those who were foreign born.

Granting that a group of academic physicians might not be representative of practitioners in general, I conducted a poll of another group of physicians, one likely to be more typical of us all, the graduates of my own class of 1958 from the State University of New York, Downstate Medical Center in Brooklyn. With this latter group, in order to draw a finer bead on how parental attitudes might affect their children's choice or rejection of medicine, I posed the question: Knowing what you do now about American medicine, if you had

Table 13.1 Physicians' Children 18 Years of Age and Older

	25 U.S. Born Parent M.D.'s	8 Other Parent M.D.'s	Total
Premedical	2	0	2
Medical students	0	1	1
Applied/rejected from medical school	1	0	1
M.D.'s	4	3	7
None of above	61	16	77
Total children	68	20	88

it to do all over again would you still choose this as a career? The possible replies were:

Yes, Probably Yes, Don't know, Probably No, and No.

First, here are the medical school results. My personal attempt at polling convinced me of at least one thing: the question that burned so brightly in my own breast was hardly a flicker in those of so many others at our school. Of the 250 faculty polled, only about one-third (87: 66 men and 21 women) bothered to respond, and only 33 of these had children eighteen and older, and thus of a suitable age for analysis. Although the sample is small and susceptible to many criticisms of a statistical nature, I refused to be undone by a p value and invite you to scan Table 13.1. Although the number of respondents was small, they turned out to be a remarkably fecund bunch. Discounting children under eighteen years of age, these 33 provided data for 88 children, an average of 2.7 per colleague.

Among the 88 children tabulated only 11 or 12.5 percent have shown any interest whatsoever in medicine, with the percentage higher among the children of foreign born parents (4/20 or 20 percent in the small sample obtained).

Among my classmates from Downstate, the response was similarly underwhelming with only 61 responses, less than half of the 150 physicians contacted. Of these 61 physicians, 3 were childless while the rest proved just as fertile as the medical school parent sample, also with 2.7 children on the average. The results of this polling, in Table 13.2, suggests that parental attitudes toward medicine can affect the career choices of their offspring.

Table 13.2 Parental Attitudes in Class of 1958 (N = 58) and Children's Choice of Medicine

Enter Medicine Again?	Any Children in Medicine?	
	Yes	No
Yes or probably yes (N = 40)	11	29
Don't know (N = 6)	3	3
No or probably no (N = 12)	1	11

No matter how well intentioned or suggestive such personal polling may turn out to be, what we are really interested in are national trends in the desirability of medicine as a profession. There are about a half million physicians among the 250 million or more American citizens. Where are our current doctors coming from and how might this affect the future of American medicine?

A much more reliable source for such information than Dr. Weisse's Personal Polling Service is the Association of American Medical Colleges. Each year it collects all kinds of information about applicants to medical school and about those who finally matriculate. The story regarding the size of the applicant pool is pretty clear. A peak occurred in 1974 with 42,624 applicants. Then there followed a precipitous decline over the next fourteen years with the nadir of 26,721 reached in 1988. The reasons for this may be argued, but more important, in terms of the present discussion, is the sharp upturn over subsequent years with a record making number of 46,968 applicants in 1995, according to their latest published results (1996).

Even more relevant to our question is the parental occupations reported by those applying to medical school over this span of years. According to the Association of American Medical Colleges, between 1981 and 1990, physician fathers constituted a steady 10.0 to 10.4 percent among the nearly 126,000 applicants queried. Mother-physicians rose from 0.8 percent to 1.5 percent, no doubt reflecting the increasing percentage of older women physicians over the last twenty years. By 1994 the total number of physician-parents rose to 18.6 percent (15.8 percent fathers and 2.8 percent mothers). So, according to this data, if anything, there seems to have been an increasing trend of medical parental connection among applicants for the last decade and a half, despite the crescendo of moans and groans emanating from such parents about the changing status of their profession during the same period.

Perhaps the situation is not so bleak as initially suggested by the New Jersey Medical School in Newark.

An additional question that might be posed about all this is whether there is any gain to having the medical torch passed from physician fathers and mothers to their sons and daughters. My gut feeling is that in general there is not. I doubt that most of the medical greats of the past inherited their profession as part of a family tradition, despite some prominent lines established within this context in the past. The precise genealogy of medical genius would be an interesting study to perform, but one that is still waiting in the wings as far as this writer is aware.

Whatever the true nature of all these considerations, the fact remains that in the Weisse household, despite a constant barrage of enthusiasm about the joys and satisfactions of medicine, neither of our children is following in our footsteps (even though the veterinarian comes close).

So why do I continue my ludicrously nonproductive habit of coin hoarding? Perhaps it is just a reflection of my childhood piggy bank obsession. Or perhaps there lurks a more substantial reason. After all, down the line we can be expecting grandchildren. . . .

14

A Sin for Saint William?

THE MEDICAL PROFESSION is seldom quick to heap praise upon one of its own. Perhaps it is because we are always seeing people at their worst, since we attend them almost exclusively during illness when human frailty is all too evident. Or it might be the knowledge of our own limitations, the knowledge that, eventually, we have no choice but to fail our patients since they all must die despite our finest efforts.

In relatively modern times the most outstanding exception to this rule of restraint is undoubtedly William—later Sir William—Osler (1849–1919). Whenever physicians wish to exemplify some paragon of medical virtue, it is his name that most readily comes to mind. It is a tribute to Osler's greatness that even during his own lifetime, it was well recognized. In 1896, one of a series of cartoon-like drawings about the Johns Hopkins Hospital depicted Osler as an archangel in heavenly robes, wings and all, riding a cyclone above the hospital from which all sorts of bacteria seemed to be taking flight. And even now, more than a half century after his death, at least a score of articles will appear each year in the medical journals, all purporting to reveal yet another admirable facet of this remarkable physician's character or accomplishments.

The outlines of the career are well known: Born in Canada, he graduated from McGill Medical School in 1872, spent two years studying in Europe, and then returned as a lecturer to McGill. In 1884 he was appointed Clinical Professor of Medicine at the University of Pennsylvania and five years later moved to head the Department of Medicine at Johns Hopkins where he became known as one of the "Big Four" who created the superb institution that continues to bear their mark. (The others were Welch in pathology, Halsted in surgery, and Kelly in gynecology.) In 1905 Osler was appointed Regius Professor of Medicine at Oxford, England, and was made a baronet in 1911.

Throughout his professional life, he contributed most by his own example.

At a time when little could be done for an illness but observe it, Osler was the most acute, persistent, and intelligent of observers. He combined his knowledge of pathology and clinical medicine in a number of papers and a famous textbook that had numerous editions. He popularized the bedside teaching method with students and house officers, and this continues to be the mainstay of clinical instruction throughout most of the world.

To read about him now, one could easily gain the impression that there was no imperfection in his teachings, no blemish to the legacy that he left us. Osler, of course, would have been the first to disagree. Originally intended for the ministry, he retained throughout his life a philosophical bent. Much more than most physicians of his time, he was deeply steeped in the classics, and his erudition in this area later earned him the singular distinction of being chosen as president of the British Classical Association. Despite the adulation he received from his contemporaries, he never lost the ability to stand off from himself, as it were, and make objective observations.

It is in this spirit that we should consider what were some rather unusual ideas for Osler's time, ideas on the aging process and its impact on a person's intellectual vitality. He broached this subject in one of a series of lectures he delivered at Johns Hopkins toward the end of his career and which were later collected and published. It was in the talk entitled "The Fixed Period" that he said:

> I am going to be very bold and touch upon another question of some delicacy, but of infinite importance in university life: one that has not been settled in this country. I refer to a fixed period for the teacher, either of time of service or of age. . . . I have two fixed ideas well known to my friends, harmless obsessions with which I sometimes bore them, but which have a direct bearing on this important problem. The first is the comparative uselessness of men above forty years of age. . . . The effective, moving, vitalizing work of the world is done between the ages of twenty-five and forty. . . . Vesalius, Harvey, Hunter, Bichat, Laennec, Virchow, Lister, Koch—the green years were yet upon their heads when their epoch-making studies were made. . . .
> My second fixed idea is the uselessness of men above sixty years of age and the incalculable benefit it would be in commercial, political and in professional life if, as a matter of course, men stopped work at this age. . . . As it can be maintained that all the great advances have come from men under forty, so the history of the world shows that a large proportion of the evils may be traced to the sexagenarians.[1]

Although Osler touched upon Anthony Trollope's suggestion for chloroform at this juncture, he hesitated at heartily endorsing it "as my own time is getting short."

Why was Osler so hard on advancing age? Perhaps he had become increasingly aware of his own failing powers as death approached or at least observed this in his patients. Certainly at the turn of the century, health and social conditions being what they were, most men past the age of forty were probably a good deal older biologically than their counterparts today. Furthermore, during Osler's time the number of full-time teachers of medicine were few, and he was properly concerned about their being allowed to vegetate in positions of academic power with no opportunity for the infusion of new blood at the top. Even today in many countries the "Herr Professor" tradition is maintained, and only death seems able to vacate major chairs in the various departments.

How much substance was there to Osler's reasoning? No doubt a preponderant number of new ideas do come from those who are not yet beyond the age of forty, but with infectious diseases essentially uncontrolled until the twentieth century, many acknowledged giants in science and art never lived to see the age of fifty. Laennec, Cohnheim, Paracelsus, Schubert, Keats, Mozart, and others like them died before completion of the fifth decade of life. Who is to say what they might or might not have accomplished in their later years had they lived? One might also point out that Harvey was fifty years of age when he completed his famous treatise on the circulation of the blood and then went on in later life at the age of seventy-three to publish in defense of the 72-page treatise a 500-page compendium which also included a vast array of information on a wide range of other biological and medical phenomena. Darwin was fifty-nine when he published *The Origin of Species* and sixty-two when he produced *The Descent of Man*. Pasteur was forty-three when he first began his investigations on the disease of silkworms and then accomplished his magnificent work on anthrax, chicken cholera, and rabies, the latter at sixty-three. The famed cardiologist Sir James Mackenzie did not even begin his monumental polygraphic studies on irregularities of the pulse until past forty years of age. In the arts, Michelangelo, Picasso, Stravinsky, and Milhaud were still exploring new possibilities in painting and music well into their eighties, and Verdi produced perhaps his most sublime opera, *Falstaff*, in his eightieth year.

Thus far we have only considered the innovative aspect of human accomplishment, in sum total a small, albeit infinitely precious, particle. It's true that the rare insight of genius may shed light on the paths we are to follow, but it remains for the mundane daily endeavors of the rest of us to lubricate the wheels of progress along them. Every great discovery has required in its wake the proselytizers and pragmatists to incorporate it into our civilization. Darwin needed his Huxley and Freud his own disciples. The roles of the great teachers, as well, cannot be overemphasized. In physiology, for example, in the late nineteenth century, many of the important discoveries could be traced to members of Carl Ludwig's institute in Leipzig where his benign, intelligent, and enthusiastic personality provided the intellectual climate in which new ideas could be tested, and youthful investigators could be allowed to spread their wings. Max Born, no doubt, performed a similar service for physics in Gottingen during the 1920s.

The idea of structuring our society on some concept of a "fixed period" for this or that not only ignores individual variation but, more importantly, the simple fact that for most of us, neither before nor after forty will the great idea come. No matter how hard we work and how well-intentioned our objectives, in the world of ideas, the overwhelming preponderance of us are essentially drones. Meanwhile, the outstanding minds among us are so few that it is unlikely that they will be overlooked.

Inasmuch as Osler influenced the thinking of so many generations of physicians and, in turn, their patients, to what extent, we must ask, have his views on aging been realized in the fabric of our present life? Witness our current youth-obsessed culture with its forty-five year olds almost officially dubbed "has-beens," and its sixty-five year olds who, for all intents and purposes, are considered "never-weres." To what extent could the "harmless obsession" of Osler have contributed to this?

Oddly enough, Osler himself, for all his great contributions to clinical medicine, teaching, and medical administration, could not be called a great scientific innovator. He was not an experimenter and made no singular major discovery with the exception of, perhaps, one. In a series of communications, culminating in one entitled, "On the Visceral Manifestations of the Erythema Group of Skin Diseases,"[2] he pointed out that what had previously been considered exclusively in the realm of dermatology were actually superficial manifestations of widespread systemic disorders. This report is believed to have stimulated the whole development of the study of connective tissue diseases, a major area of intense investigation up to the present. He was fifty-five at the time.

Notes

1. Osler W. *Aequanimitas with Other Addresses to Medical Students, Nurses, and Practitioners of Medicine*, 2nd ed. Philadelphia, Pa.: Blakiston, 1928, 397–400.
2. Osler W. On the visceral manifestations of the erythema group of skin diseases. Am J Med Sci 1904; 128:1–25.

15

In the Service of the IRS

LIKE ANY OTHER red-blooded American, I want as little to do with the Internal Revenue Service as is humanly possible. But when this arm of our government calls for your help in retrieving millions of dollars that some nefarious plotters have excluded from our treasury, who can resist this appeal to patriotism? Certainly not I, and when the call came to me, I was soon knee deep in the controversy surrounding the alleged scam.

The genesis of the case was actually more than two world wars ago. Shortly before the outbreak of hostilities between the United States and Germany in World War I, a major German industrial giant, fearful of having its substantial American holdings confiscated, turned them all over to an employee who was a faithful American national but who, in the final analysis, could also be relied upon to do his duty for the parent company. At the conclusion of the war in 1918 when these holdings were turned back to the German company, their American agent was rewarded for his stalwart performance with large chunks of stock, the basis for his family's fortune.

The only son and heir of this man was as astute and hard working as his father and managed to increase the family's wealth even more, aided in part by the effect of economic trends over the next thirty or forty years. As he continued to amass enormous wealth, he waited until middle age before acquiring someone to share it with him, oddly enough a simple American farm girl, far removed from the opulent kind of existence that had always surrounded her husband. Her down-home direct approach to life, unaffected by all the trappings of wealth, never deserted her and was a distinct part of her charm and attraction as she filled her husband's home with several children before he passed on many years before her.

As the sole heir to his fortune, the youngish widow never remarried but instead devoted herself to her children and grandchildren for the many remaining years of her life. It was an uninterrupted robust one until her early seventies when she developed a serious condition that affected one of her heart valves, aortic stenosis. It soon became necessary for open-heart surgery to be undertaken, and the diseased valve was replaced with a mechanical prosthesis.

Soon after the successful surgery, she began to divest herself of large portions of her wealth, transferring it to her daughters and sons who were now in their forties and fifties and already with children of their own entered into adulthood. By the time the elderly lady finally did succumb to her heart disease seven years post surgery, all but a fraction of her former fortune was now in the hands of her surviving children.

The U.S. government's contention was that this transfer of wealth on the part of the widow was a deliberate scheme to avoid estate taxes in the face of her realization that only a few years of life would be left to her following such a major operation in a person of her advanced age. The family's defense against this charge was that their mother and grandmother had no anticipation at all of dying so soon after her successful heart surgery. Aside from the valve problem, her health had always been unusually good. The surgery and its aftermath had gone smoothly, and all the symptoms that had precipitated the need for surgery in the first place had disappeared rapidly postoperatively. Her own mother had lived until the age of ninety-six, and her family indicated that the old lady at their head, following replacement of the defective valve, had every intention of doing the same if not even bettering the record.

The reason for her breaking up the family fortune, they maintained, was that she realized late in life that even if she was to live until the age of 106, she could never manage to spend a significant portion of her money even if she was shamefully extravagant, something which she certainly was not. Her intention in distributing her wealth when she did was to enable her children and grandchildren to enjoy it at a time in life when their own health was good and they could most enjoy the advantages of the kind of lifestyle that this money could provide.

Therefore, it was not the state of her heart that was in question, but the state of her mind as she redistributed her wealth among her progeny. So where did I come in? As an expert in cardiovascular disease, I had the job of convincing the judge that life expectancy following such surgery in an elderly person was not great and thereby support the contention of the IRS that it was to avoid taxes that the disbursement of all these funds took place at this time during the matriarch's life.

On purely scientific grounds my medical case was easily made. No matter how skillful the cardiac surgeon might be, the artificial heart valves of the time were far from ideal substitutes for our God-given natural valves. They were foreign bodies that we were inserting, and they had moving parts that could become stuck. After thousands upon thousands of heartbeats, they could break free from the moorings to which they were sutured. Blood clots tended to form on their surfaces. These or excessive scar formation over the valve surface could result in obstruction. Finally, bacteria, which are frequently released into our blood stream after dental manipulations or even vigorous tooth brushing but are routinely removed from the blood stream in normal individuals, could often find a nesting site on such artificial valves and result in life-threatening infections (prosthetic valve endocarditis).

All in all, it was estimated in one report that within five years of such valve insertions it was likely that in 50 percent of such patients, one of these devastating complications might occur, resulting in the need for risky re-operation if not the death of the patient. It was one of these complications that took the widow off so suddenly and unexpectedly.

The case was to be decided by a judge rather than jury, and prior to the court date, I met with the IRS lawyer with whom I was to prepare our presentation. The young man who visited my office immediately struck me by his close resemblance to Harvard's Alan Dershowitz, but I was soon to learn, the resemblance stopped there. Several weeks later we sat together in the courtroom having arrived a bit early to await the entrance of the opposition.

The doors at the rear of the courtroom swung open, and a phalanx of very impressive lawyers from one of the most prestigious firms in the city ceremoniously made their way down the center aisle. To say they were impressive was an understatement. Majestic came to mind, and I cocked an ear, almost expecting to hear organ music accompanying the procession. They literally gleamed in confidence and sartorial splendor. I would have ventured a guess that even their shoelaces would have outpriced the entire wardrobe of the two government representatives opposing them. Following close behind their legal champions were the family imperial, with righteous indignation inscribed on each and every countenance.

The cardiologist they had employed to represent them was a very competent one who had cared for the deceased during her final years. Not surprisingly, he was himself descended from the higher reaches of society, he and his father before him having ministered to their needs over many decades. His role was simply to testify that in his opinion, his patient had done extraordinarily well postoperatively, that her death had come as something of a surprise to him in view of her excellent response to surgery, and that despite this, she had never indicated to him in any way that she had expected anything other than a great number of years left to her following her surgical ordeal.

The medical portion of the testimony was pretty straightforward. It was on the legal side that I was sure the government's case had faltered, in no small measure, I ascertained, due to the demeanor of its legal representative. My partner was well prepared but much too tentative. He did not speak up clearly and constantly seemed obliged to refer to his notes even though I knew he had committed them to memory. In short, it was not a stellar courtroom performance.

The opposition, on the other hand, were equally well prepared but silky smooth and bursting with confidence in their convictions. Endless depositions, affidavits, and what-all were extracted from their gleaming attaché cases as they serenely laid their case before the judge. They were so adept and full of themselves that I wondered as an almost neutral observer if this might prove off-putting to the stern and laconic jurist who presided over the whole affair. For my part, I had no idea what had been in the old lady's mind as she doled out all those millions. I could easily have been persuaded that it really was the simple generosity of a loving mother and grandmother that motivated her actions in the final years of her life. Fortunately, it was not my case to decide.

The formal court presentations came to a close, and the court retired to consider the evidence. The judgment, rendered a week or so later, was that there were insufficient grounds to indicate that the woman had expected a foreshortened existence, and thus, the case was decided in favor of the family.

This did not, however, conclude my connection with the case. The judge's decision proved, on the contrary, only a stopping point along the road I was to travel with the IRS over the next year. My extended involvement with that agency hinged simply upon the fact that they seemed totally incapable of providing me with the fee specified when I agreed to testify for them.

It was not a lot of money, considering the amount of time and effort I expended, only a thousand dollars. Indeed, when I finally became aware that the sum hoped to be recovered by the government might run as high as 13 million dollars, I calculated that, had they succeeded, my "cut" would have amounted to less than eight thousandths of 1 percent. Given my sense of civic duty, I could live with this, even though the realization that the opposing lawyers and their doctor must have walked off with infinitely more could have poured salt into the wound if I chose to let it. It was the action, or rather inaction of the IRS that accomplished just this.

Three months went by with no check in the mail. I then began a round of telephone calls and correspondence to the various arms of the IRS that might have been involved, all to no avail. By the time nine months had elapsed after the decision had been handed down and I had still not been paid, I took the only other course left to me, an appeal to my congressman. He excelled at this sort of service for his constituents, and a week after my appeal, his office wrote me that they would pursue the matter. A week after this, a check for one thousand dollars arrived from the IRS. A week later, a second check for one thousand dollars arrived from the IRS.

After all the grief they had caused me, I was momentarily tempted to pocket the second check and just sit tight. Then an idea occurred to me as to how I might take one small step in the name of all those who had ever had to tangle with the IRS bureaucracy and one giant step for my own sense of self-satisfaction and fun.

I cashed the second check and issued one of my own for $910 payable to the IRS. The practice of the agency was to charge a 12 percent annual rate of interest for all money owed them and vice versa if they, perchance, had owed any money to a taxpayer. Since this amounted to a monthly charge of 1 percent on any balance, I calculated that over nine months, ninety dollars in interest had accrued to me. When I sent that check to the IRS, little did I imagine how this was to shake the U.S. Treasury to its very foundations. A flurry of telephone calls and correspondence followed in its wake, all protesting that since the contract I had signed was only for $1,000 and not $1,090, there was no possible way that the system could tolerate such a deviation.

I was unmoved by such protestations. I knew very well that every day the IRS was breaking an assumed contract—the tax code—by making all kinds of deals with defaulting screen stars, sports heroes, and Wall Street traders. Hundreds of thousands of dollars in taxpayer money had been written off in this way, not to mention the hundreds of millions we have lost to such deadbeats as Brazil and Poland, for example. In view of all this I refused to believe that my ninety dollars represented an insurmountable obstacle to the survival of the system.

Finally the kid gloves came off, and I began to receive calls and letters of a different nature. These all hinted darkly as to the possible role of the Department of Justice in my case if I did not come around. I actually warmed to the prospect of such an encounter and looked forward to the opportunity of revealing in open court how all those long distance telephone calls to me had probably already greatly exceeded the amount that they intended to recover in the first place. The time spent by secretaries and stenographers was an add-on, not even to mention the hours of wasted attorneys' time spent in pursuit of my ninety dollars. By the time the threats had begun to arrive, all those phone calls had put me and the IRS attorney who was constantly in touch with me on an almost chummy basis. I verbalized about the possibilities of my testimony and how some magazines and talk show hosts might be interested in discussing how the government's money was routinely spent in such efforts.

As I began, almost palpably, to sense a rising discomfort at the other end of the line, I played my final card. To put an end to the business once and for all, as a gesture of good faith, I would be willing to send a token sum to the IRS in settlement: five dollars. With visions of media mayhem probably dancing in his head, the lawyer replied that he would take it under advisement. A few days later his reply arrived.

"We have considered your gesture of conciliation," he wrote. "While the amount offered is not nearly as much as we had hoped, we have decided to accept your offer in the spirit in which it is made. . . . When we receive your check we will close our file on the case."

And they did.

This all happened many years ago, and I therefore am not concerned about ruffling the feathers of any individuals within the IRS by writing about it now. My erstwhile IRS colleagues have probably risen within the ranks and acquired enough mellowness to look upon this little imbroglio with almost as much amusement as I. It is equally as likely that armed with all that knowledge about the inner workings of the IRS, they have even "deserted to the enemy" and proved invaluable within the ranks of accounting and law firms devoted to protecting other family fortunes from what they might consider unjustified depredations by the U.S. government.

Still there was some trepidation on my part in putting this all down in print for anyone to see. The IRS does not shine too brightly in the reflection of the light I have chosen to cast upon it, and deserved or not, it does have a reputation for vindictiveness. We are even aware that some previous administrations have used it to settle scores with offensive or offending individuals. But this is all in the past and could never be repeated in the present.

You might ask, "What, never?"

Well, hardly ever.

16

What's in a Name?

ON JANUARY 6, 1896, the *New York Sun* informed its readers of a great new discovery by a Professor Routgen *[sic]* of Wurzburg University in Germany. A hundred years after the discovery of X Rays by Wilhelm Conrad Roentgen, I wonder if we have become any more precise in written or other, more recent, types of communication about science.

The popular *MacNeil/Lehrer News Hour* on public television (now minus MacNeil) often features an oral essay by one of their stable of gurus as an epilogue to the in-depth reporting of some of the leading news events of the day. Not long ago, one of these individuals, an earnest young woman, closed her piece with mention of that great American microbiologist, "Norman Sabin." She would have been a bit more convincing, to this viewer at least, if she had referred to the discoverer of the oral polio vaccine as the rest of us knew him, Albert B. Sabin.

Such gaffes are not limited to television newscasts. In a recent extensively researched review of the Type A personality and its possible relationship to coronary heart disease,[1] the author included fourteen publications by the originators of this hypothesis among her ninety-one references. Within the text she chose to ignore the first name of Ray Rosenman but did even worse by his colleague when she converted Meyer Friedman, the physician, into Milton Friedman, the economist.

Even one of my favorite medical writers, Richard Selzer, I found susceptible to this kind of error when, in his autobiography, *Down from Troy*, he refers to the creator of that famous nineteenth-century painting of a doctor sitting at the bedside of a critically ill patient as Lucas Fields[2] instead of Sir Samuel Luke Fildes.

Physicians and other scientists, especially, must find this disturbing. Is this a new trend, I wonder, or has such solecistic sloppiness always been in evidence, and only in my crotchety declining years am I becoming more sensitive about it? In my own case, I have good reason to be on guard against such errors, my name being a particularly troubling one. To be quite frank, I am not sure what I really should be calling myself. When my paternal grandfather, whom I never knew, arrived at Ellis Island from Bialystok, he called himself something that I believe sounded like "Vissavahter." I have divined that "vissa" probably represented a bastardization of *weiss*, German or Yiddish for "white," while "vahter" probably derived from *woda*, Polish for "water." If, in the manner of some immigrants, I ever decided to Americanize my name, I would be calling myself Allen Whitewater, an ersatz Native American if there ever was one. No matter; the immigration agent, who no doubt had just processed a boatload of Germans, shortened it to Weiss.

My father was born in Philadelphia. As a young man he moved to New York City and was shocked to find page after page of Weiss in the Manhattan telephone directory. Affronted by the prospect of being just one among so many, he later added an "e" to the end, and there it has perched precariously ever since. ("Weiss with an e at the end," has been a necessary part of every introduction for all the children and grandchildren who have fallen heirs to that alteration.)

The spelling of my first name is another fluke. "Allen" is ordinarily used as a surname. However, when as a small child in grammar school I was asked to write my name, I did so phonetically: Al-len. After all, does anyone say Al-lan or A-lan, as the more common spellings usually go? Only years later when I glanced at my birth certificate did I realize that I had saved myself from an even worse fate. I know not whether it was temporary perversity on the part of my parents or the registrar, but there it was, officially inscribed: "Alen B. Weiss." (The B is for Barry, by the way, a sort of sissy middle name I never quite cared for as a boy.)

We Americans are a casual lot; we often start calling each other by first names after only the briefest of acquaintances, something which I was not brought up to do and therefore resist. We also tend to contract difficult names into more manageable shorthand forms at every opportunity. With the large number of foreign born physicians on our hospital staffs, I have noted the nurses to be particularly adept at the art of abbreviated identification. Doctors Ravindranathan, Dasmahapatra, and Tiruviluamala quickly become Doctors Ravi, Das, and Tiru in the nurses' efforts to keep their tongues untied.

In the past, some have succumbed to other pressures of Americanization in altering their names. When I discover a Cohen who has been converted to

What's in a Name?

Crane, a Darechinsky to a Darrin, a Ruggiero to a Rogers, or a Carbone to a Cole, I wonder a little sadly whether efforts at camouflage were also intended.

Not so for many Greek-Americans, though. Papadopoulos, just in case you did not know, means "son of the priest." So when you meet a Pappas, you are, symbolically at least, dealing with the priesthood. And all those Poulos's are "sons of" something or other but undeniably still proud Hellenes.

Despite the pressures, not to mention the convenience, of name changing, I am personally drawn to those who have chosen not to reject their original identities. An old colleague of mine, a very short Greek with a very long name, Anagnostopoulos (son of the reader), has kept it inviolate. Those long Polish names, the kind with fourteen consonants without a vowel in sight to guide you through them, can be the most perplexing. Yet many Polish-Americans doggedly hold on to them for dear life. I do know one who has called a sort of truce in this battle. His name is Adam Hyrniewicki, daunting despite the obvious vowels present. He has offered us a way out by inserting "Smith" in between for the faint hearted. As a token of respect, though, I choose to use his last name, pronounced hernia-vitzky, easy for a doctor to remember.

There are some guardians of their identity I admire even more. In the post–World War II years, Adolf was not exactly the most popular name to have in these parts. Yet one of the most gentle and decent people I have helped train, a German immigrant, explained to me that it was not of his choosing that his father had so named him but that out of respect for his father, he would keep it. An earlier Adolf was unfortunate enough to have a family name from which our own "improper" verb for sexual intercourse derives from the German. But Adolf Fick (1829–1901) stuck with it, and all those of us who use his principle for the calculation of cardiac output or mention other accomplishments of this outstanding physicist have done so for years without even the faintest trace of a snicker, a credit to his and his family's fortitude.

My favorite story about names concerns a family that had immigrated here from Eastern Europe. The closest one can come to pronouncing their name in English is Koven. The official who confronted it at Ellis Island, obviously a son of Erin, did not quite hear it that way and, perhaps with a little twinkle in his eye, wrote down "Quinn."

One of the family labelled thus, the great uncle of the man who related the story to me, agonized over what he considered an abomination of his family name by this ill-fitting and unwanted disguise. After years of being identified as Mr. Quinn, he went to court and legally had it changed back to Koven. In succeeding years, whenever asked about this, the old man would respond in an unmistakable Russo-Yiddish accent that perhaps only in China could be mistaken for a brogue, "I didn't want people to think that I was trying to pass as Irish."

Owen H. Wangensteen (1898–1981), who headed the Department of Surgery at the University of Minnesota for thirty-seven years and knew just about everyone who was anyone in the field during that time, had more than just a passing acquaintance with the famous Mayo brothers. He was closer to Doctor Will and once recalled to me, "Will Mayo remembered everybody; Charles Mayo remembered nobody. His wife asked him once who he was having for dinner and he said, 'My chief resident, but I don't recall his name.'"

I must confess that despite all my carrying on about names, I am more like Charles than William Mayo in this respect, and I am a little ashamed of it.

All this, as you no doubt have already surmised, is not only about scientific accuracy and proper referencing. There is something more human and caring about a person who not only remembers your name but also gets it right.

From here on out, I am going to try harder at it.

Notes

1. Lachar BL. Coronary-prone behavior: type A behavior revisited. Texas Heart Inst J 1993; 20:143–151.

2. Selzer R. *Down from Troy: A Doctor Comes of Age.* Boston: Back Bay Books, 1992, 125.

17

PC

Politically Correct or Potentially Corrupting?

WHAT IS WRONG with the title, "Isolated Left Main Coronary Ostial Stenosis in Oriental People" that appeared in a medical journal in 1993?

Many of you will probably object to the term Oriental, but before you do, let me provide some additional information: the authors are Koh, Hwang, Kim, Lee, Kyoon, Lim, Han, Lee, Park, and Yoon; the study emanated from a university hospital in Korea; and the editors of the *Journal of the American College of Cardiology* had the uncommon good sense to leave it alone.

All of which brings me to a trend that some of us find silly, insidious, dishonest, and, ultimately, infuriating: the use of so-called "politically correct" jargon for descriptions of racial and religious groups, jargon that has become increasingly overbearing.

Not long ago I distributed a confidential questionnaire to a class of medical students at my school. Anonymity was provided the responders so that they might not feel inhibited in any way in their replies to the questions posed. Among other items, a question of identity based on race was included. However, after the terms indicating white, African-American, and Hispanic, I was a little stumped when it came to the Asian continent. Because of the wide diversity of the racial mix contained within it, I listed "Oriental" and then "Other" to help sort them out a bit as well as provide an entry space for Native Americans and any others accidentally overlooked.

It turned out that among the 150 students polled, about a quarter could trace their ancestries to Asia, and of these, about half could be identified as Indian in origin. What I was not prepared for was the response of about a half dozen of those with Asian backgrounds to the use of the term "Oriental." Notations on the questionnaire advised me to "get with it," stop using racial epithets, with one instructing me that "Oriental" was a term that could only be applied to inanimate objects such as furniture and not people.

To someone who has always admired Far Eastern art, culture, and food, it came as something of a shock to learn that all this time I had really been a racial bigot: I, who have considered it my good fortune to have spent a good chunk of my life in big cities that contained large Chinatowns (Asian-American towns?); one whose home is adorned with many representations of Far Eastern art; and one who has joked about moving to the suburbs only when a town was found with over a half-dozen Chinese restaurants and two Indian ones practically within walking distance, and, yes, one who considers members of a wide diversity of racial and religious groups within the circle of his dearest friends.

It is true that nearly a hundred years ago in pulp fiction, characters like Dr. Fu Manchu may have been referred to as "inscrutable Orientals," but unlike "yellow," as in "yellow peril" and similar racial slurs, "Oriental," I contend, remains a useful and nonpejorative term to describe Chinese, Japanese, Koreans, Thais, and residents of what was once called French Indochina. To simply label them as Asians and then include the native populations of India and the Philippines, for example, under this heading would hardly be edifying to any demographer or other kind or researcher attempting to seek patterns of illness, behavior, or belief based on racial origin and diverse cultures.

Lumping all those with Asian roots under the heading of "Asian-American," is as useful as including everyone from the Isthmus of Panama to the Arctic Ocean within the category of "North Americans."

The problem of racial and ethnic identification does not end there. Perhaps among no minority has the choice of proper nomenclature proved such a challenge as for those originally transported here from Africa as slaves. It is understandable from the point of view of the Civil Rights movement that older terms with negative connotations were rejected by the activists of the sixties and thereafter.

"Negro" and "colored" were too tied to the past that many were struggling to escape or overcome. Gradually "black" became the term of preference. I must admit not understanding the thrust of "black is beautiful" at first—all races have their ugly ones of course—but, in retrospect, it was an inspirational idea. Throughout the language "black" carried with it so many negative undertones: black hearted, blackball, black mood, black mark, blackguard, and so on. By stressing a positive, even idealized use of the term, people gradually denuded it of such unwarranted meanings and "black" became a respectable term for race, unencumbered by its former linguistic burdens. Both blacks and nonblacks finally came to use it comfortably. That is until "African-American" came along.

Perhaps it was inevitable that as we became more and more aware that Americans are more of a potpourri than a melting pot, we came to accept the many distinctive ingredients that maintained each ethic group's original character throughout. Ethnicity became the vogue and identification by hyphenation all the rage. After Greek- Italian- Irish- and German- among others, African- could be considered a natural development.

Although I will gladly address members of any racial or ethnic group by precisely the term they prefer, in this instance I am inclined to "black" rather than "African-American" because I believe that the strength of good prose lies in its sinews of simple and direct language whenever this is possible. In this respect "black" wins hands down over the somewhat cumbersome "African-American." (I readily admit that I do not think twice about "Italian-American," for example, but hasten to add that if there were a shorter, nonobjectionable term available, I would unhesitatingly use it.)

In the final analysis, though, African-American poses no interpretive problems. Classification of African-Africans, on the other hand, presents innumerable ones. To the casual observer, Somalis and Ethiopians might seem closely related ethnically as well as geographically, but among each group there are probably many who would find objections to such a grouping, and both would have obvious grounds for refusing to be lumped along with the inhabitants of Ghana or Zambia, for example, simply as Africans.

The Arab peoples of the north can certainly be distinguished from the black Africans of middle and southern Africa, and even within a single country such as Egypt, the Nubians in the south are undoubtedly different from their countrymen in the north.

Getting back to the United States and current practices here, pussy footing around about such terminology suggests to me in itself an inherent manifestation of racism, a reflection of discomfort about being honest and precise in one's descriptions or classifications. The Australian-born critic, Robert Hughes, in his book, *Culture of Complaint: The Fraying of America*, observes, "Just as language grotesquely inflates in attack, so it timidly shrinks in approbation, seeking words that cannot possibly give any offense, however notational. We do not fail, we underachieve. We are not junkies, but substance abusers; not handicapped, but differently abled." Learning of a suggestion in one of our medical journals that a corpse should be referred to as "a nonliving person," Hughes acerbically comments that perhaps, by extension, a fat corpse should be called "a differently sized nonliving person."[1]

"Caucasian" is a favorite of the politically correct although it makes me, for one, bristle. Agreed that "white" does not accurately describe all the shades from gray to ruddy red that also characterize those of basically European extraction, everybody at least understands what the term includes. To suggest that all such come from a mountainous region in southeastern Europe is preposterous, and to use this for "white" makes this observer see red.

Euphemisms have often represented ill-disguised hostility. In the past whenever those of the Jewish faith heard themselves referred to as "Hebrews" or "Israelites" by gentiles in positions of power, it is understandable how they might have felt a strong urge to run for cover to a civil rights lawyer or to another admissions or employment office.

Today the pendulum on religious viewpoint has swung completely the other way. "Judeo-Christian" is still pretty much in favor in describing generally how Americans feel on ethical and moral issues, but given the widening scope of religious beliefs among our citizenry, it is running the risk of rapidly becoming not politically correct. The redoubtable satirist, Art Buchwald, not long ago did a piece on the Judeo-Christian ethic. Tongue in cheek, he raised questions about the criminal omission of other religious segments in our society and wound up suggesting a more appropriate term, something along the lines of Judeo-Christian-Islamic-Hindu-atheistic-agnostic-Zoroastrian to fit the bill.

There seems to be no end to the number of controversies raging now about such questions of terminology. Hispanics/Latinos are engaged in their own internecine dispute as to what they want to be called, and so this outside observer will have to pass.

"So what does all this have to do with medicine?" you might well ask.

In recent years it has struck me as I have perused case reports in various journals that the racial description of the patient is often omitted. Similarly, when groups of patients with a particular disease or syndrome are reported, there is no racial breakdown, contrary to good epidemiological practice. Surely there can be no disagreement about the frequent importance of race in relative resistance or susceptibility to certain diseases. Then why leave out such important information?

Let us take this a few steps further. What about religion? Would not someone identified as a Seventh Day Adventist or Latter Day Saint convey something to you regarding the little likelihood of alcoholism as a contributing factor to his or her complaint? Might not the potential modes of therapy be influenced by religious beliefs of a Jehovah's Witness or a Christian Scientist?

What about occupation? This is recognized as a critical bit of information that might clue one in to the possibility of a variety diseases more likely to occur in farmers, coal miners, construction workers, chemists, and others with well-known risky industrial or environmental exposure. But there is valuable information to be gained from knowledge of employment history of just about all patients. If, for example, you knew the patient was a business executive or college professor, you would rarely be amiss in your reliance on their recounting of their past medical history and the patient's understanding of the illness, its treatment, and prognosis than might be the case were the patient holding a job not even requiring a high school diploma. Despite the usefulness of such data, I find it is like digging a tunnel through a mountainside with a pickax to get such information from house staff and medical students.

The trouble is that collectively, we are all so intent on being politically correct that we become guilty of becoming scientifically and morally *incorrect*. I am reminded of an instance some years ago when a major governmental institution erected a large new building in the midst of an economically depressed area containing many Hispanics. Within it, on the doors of all the rest rooms they added "Caballeros" or "Senoras" to "Men" and "Women." As if Spanish-speaking people, even poor and uneducated ones, could not figure this out for themselves without such a crutch. Needless to add, such a gesture was unaccompanied by specific actions that might have improved the social, economic, or health status of the Hispanics within that community. To quote Robert Hughes again, "No shifting of words is going to reduce the amount of bigotry in this or any other society."[2]

The hypocrisy of which he writes suffuses all such linguistic artifices. Instead of being so intent on being politically correct, perhaps it is time to recognize that it is more important to be honest, caring, and forthright if we are truly to fulfill our roles as healers, patient advocates, and simply good citizens.

Notes

1. Hughes R. *Culture of Complaint: The Fraying of America*. New York: Oxford Univ. Press, 1993, 20.

2. Hughes, 21.

18

SI Units

Wrong for the Right Reasons

I WAS LOST in Amsterdam. My first visit to "The Venice of the North," and after hours of entranced wandering across countless little bridges over equally many small canals, I had no idea of where I was. Dusk had suddenly come upon the city, and just about all the inhabitants, who seemingly moments before had crowded the streets, had disappeared into their homes. Or so it seemed in the backwater alley where I now found myself.

But then I spied some hope of assistance. Before me there stood on the edge of the canal a two or three story tower. A light that showed through a window up top indicated that someone was inside, and the entrance door was ajar. I entered tentatively and mounted the winding stairs to the attic of the turret-like structure. There sat an elderly Dutchman, absentmindedly cutting away at a stick of wood with his pen knife, the shavings piling up on the floor before him.

His gaze rose momentarily, taking notice of another presence in the room.

"Excuse me, sir," I began hopefully, "but do you speak English?" No response.

My knowledge of other languages was limited but perhaps sufficient enough to understand directions back to my hotel if we hit upon a common one.

"Parlez-vous Francais?" Again no response.

"Sprechen Sie Deutsch?" Nein.

"Habla Usted Español?" Nada.

"Parla Italiano?" Niente.

He remained inside himself, apparently oblivious to me, before he broke into a broad smile, his eyes lighting up as they met mine. "Esperanto?"

The year was 1954.

For those of us old enough to remember, Esperanto was the utopian answer to the Babel of languages that had evolved throughout the world over the last few millennia. It is an artificial language invented in 1887 by, perhaps not surprisingly, a Pole. Dr. Ludwik Zamenhof, an ophthalmologist from Byalystok, concocted it, basing it mainly on Romance languages, primarily Spanish. He published his guide to the new universally proposed tongue in 1905 and became known to much of the world at large as Dr. Esperanto.

According to the *Encyclopaedia Britannica*, Dr. Esperanto has given us a run for our money. As recently as the 1970s, and perhaps into the 1980s, there were estimated to be over one hundred thousand users of Esperanto in eighty-three countries worldwide. There were also twenty-two international groups dedicated to Esperanto with over twelve hundred local clubs and societies. World Congresses on it had been held. But I ask you, "Do you know *anyone* who has ever studied Esperanto?"

In science, particularly, the need for clarity and precision in written communication is important in the interests of international understanding. The scientific counterpart to the more generally applied Esperanto was called Interlingua and was invented in 1903 by a mathematician, Giuseppe Flexione. Latin based, it read a lot like Esperanto, by which I mean essentially Spanish with a lot of "k's" and a few other novel twists thrown in. In past issues of some medical journals, I can recall summaries in Interlingua at the end of each article, but this practice seems to have been discontinued over the last ten or twenty years. I decided to check it out.

I strolled over to our medical library, and in a random way, attempting not to identify the titles of the bound volumes, picked out fifty different current journals from A to Z, after discarding any state or other local journals inadvertently selected. In none of them was there a summary in Interlingua or any other substitute international lingo.

By chance some foreign journals happened to be selected, and following the initial selection process, I went back to look into this further. I found that among the dozen or so with the designation "European" in the title, all but one were printed exclusively in English. The exception had summaries in French and German at the end of each article. The Canadians, in obvious deference to their internal ethnic strife, print both in English and French. The Scandinavians print exclusively in English.

Like it or not, English has become, in essence, the universal language of science.

All of which brings us to the subject of the title, the Systeme International (SI) Units for the expression of laboratory values in clinical medicine. It was first introduced in Europe, and from the name, the French undoubtedly had an important role in developing it.

The thrust of the new system was to convert the expression of various laboratory values from mass units (e.g., milligrams, grams) to those (e.g., millimoles, moles) more precisely reflecting the metabolic or chemical activity of the substance involved.

This logical line of reasoning, along with a desire for worldwide uniformity and understanding, along with other, more esoteric, considerations, was unassailably on good scientific grounds, and by the mid-seventies in the United States, influential editors of scholarly journals and leaders in clinical pathology and laboratory science were urging adoption of the system here. Research journals, much to the chagrin of some of us churning out material for them, began to reject all manuscripts not expressing their findings in SI Units. Pressure from on high to conform has persisted ever since.

Meanwhile, "down in the trenches" among the medical practitioners responsible for dealing more directly with patients and each other, the idea that they had been handed the Holy Grail of medical communication eluded them, despite glowing reports from influential quarters about how well the system was being accepted elsewhere and how well it was working. Frankly, back home it seemed to be sowing more confusion than enlightenment in their daily practice of medicine.

First off, they were being asked to forget all those normal values they had spent a lifetime committing to memory as they attempted to determine whether their patients were in good chemical equilibrium or in trouble. Many, if not most, could not see any deficiencies in the units they were using and what real advantages new units would provide. Certain specialists made pleas for the retention of certain of the older values for reasons they felt specifically germane to their own types of practice. Perhaps even more important than all this was the feeling of how much harm might be done to all our efforts in patient education about their health. For example, after decades of convincing them that it was in their best interests to get their cholesterols down to 200 or less (milligrams per deciliter) we would now be switching this to 5.2 (moles per liter). And for what?

This tug of war has gone on for nearly two decades without clear resolution. While awaiting it, one is prompted to become philosophical about the urge for standardization or uniformity that seems to overcome us every so often. There are always pluses and minuses along the way.

To dwell on language a bit longer, diversity often enriches rather than deprives our sensibilities. If English has become the language of science, Spanish is the lover's tongue, French that of haute cuisine, and Italian the ideal vocal expression of grand opera. On the other hand, on a foggy night with zero visibility as my jumbo jet approaches the airport on radar, I take a good deal of comfort in the knowledge that the pilot in the cockpit and the traffic controllers on the ground are communicating clearly and concisely in English and nothing else.

Money is no small consideration in such matters. In the United Kingdom, for example, the conversion of their monetary system to simple metrics, each pound now having one hundred pence, put them in step with the rest of the modern world. There were few tears shed over the loss of the old shillings, guineas, crowns, and the brain busting way change for purchases was once calculated in merry olde England. While the British took this step with relative alacrity, they wouldn't dream of conforming with the rest of the world in the way the traffic on their highways is directed. True, if they suddenly decided to drive on the right side of the road, some of us who heretofore were foolhardy enough to attempt playing switch when we drove there might now have a much easier time of it. In the process, however, who knows how many Brits might be killed or maimed by suddenly trying to drive in the "wrong" direction.

Many years ago it was determined that the traditional positioning of letters on the typewriter keyboard was inappropriate for the most efficient and rapid typing. Some letters used in the greatest abundance were not as advantageously placed as others much less frequently employed. How inefficient! No doubt somebody wanted to change it, but this never happened. Such an innovation might have paid off eventually with future generations of typists learning a new, improved system. Meanwhile it would have caused utter mayhem among those already trained in the traditional manner, not to mention disruptions resulting in the business machine industry. Meanwhile, the introduction of word processors and computers have probably speeded up the typing process infinitely more than any discombobulating revision of keyboard organization ever could for future typists.

The loss of the geographically based telephone exchange was unquestionably unavoidable given the explosion of demand for new numbers. But for some of us, there remains an irresistible nostalgia for what once was. Recall Glen Miller's classic "Pennsylvania 6–5000," and you will know why "763–5000" was never written. A fond farewell to "Pennsylvania," "Bryant," "Trafalgar," "Gramercy," and all the rest.

Zip Codes were also probably inevitable although I am convinced that no innovation will ever eliminate the incompetence of the U.S. Postal Service, not even the extra four numbers after the Zip that they want us to include and which I, for one, never will.

Viewed against this broad background, the controversy over SI Units can be seen as a paradigm, one involving rationality, regimentation, and reason. It has pitted an elite few against a reluctant majority in this country with an essential stalemate resulting.

Now in certain circles "elite" has become a dirty word, but it certainly should have no negative connotation in the realm of science. To whom if not the elite, the best minds, should we turn for guidance in such matters? On the other hand "elite" is not synonymous with "infallible," any more than knowledge necessarily connotes wisdom. And if the issue has not been decided over the last twenty years please note that the sky has not fallen.

In regard to the SI issue, our own elite, to their credit, have begun to show signs of such recognition and seem to be shifting from the purely rational track onto one of reason. Some of them at least have acknowledged that this task they once set before them with such fervor might not, in the long run, have been worth all the furor and confusion it has aroused. They have even acknowledged that perhaps elsewhere in the world, the system has not been as wholeheartedly accepted as once reported. Perhaps, finally, they have realized that if a cure for AIDS suddenly appears or a sensational new chemical for cancer treatment, whatever the units in which they are dispensed and in whatever units their effects are measured, they will be welcomed all over the world in whatever units just happen to exist in each locality.

It is in the light of this realization that the *New England Journal of Medicine*, in its July 2, 1992, issue, announced editorially its "Retreat from SI Units." In a less bold but nonetheless significant modification of policy, another influential journal, the *Annals of Internal Medicine*, announced its decision to include inserts with conversions between SI and the older standard units in all future articles published.

Through all this "sturm und drang," I could not help recalling that punch line from the show-stopping tune, "If I Were a Rich Man," sung by the character Tevye in *Fiddler on the Roof*. However, I thought of different lyrics the character might use in addressing his maker: "Would it spoil some vast eternal plan were I not an SI man?"

Obviously not.

19

The Long and the Short and the Rest of It

> Short people got no reason
> Short people got no reason
> Short people got no reason to live.
> They got little hands and little eyes,
> They walk around tellin' great big lies.
> They got little noses and little tiny teeth.
> They wear platform shoes on their nasty little feet.
> Well I don't want no short people, don't want no short people,
> Don't want no short people round here.[1]

WHEN RANDY NEWMAN wrote this ditty back in 1977, a putdown of short people was probably the last thing he had in mind. It was much more likely that he was taking a swipe at those in the majority who unfairly derogate those among us who just happen to fail in matching whatever society considers the norm. Misguided outrage throughout the country led to suppression of the song and its elimination from the airways, marking Newman as one of the earliest victims of the nascent political correctness movement.

As a lifelong "vertically challenged person," myself, I was not at all offended by the song. I thought it funny as well as meaningful then and now. I still chuckle over the lyrics when I read them. It is true, however, that short people are often short changed by height-obsessed American society. Tall men have always had the upper hand (pun intended). I can well recall as a boy seeing on the silver screen that pulchritudinous piranha of femininity, Mae West, issuing an invitation to "Come up and see me sometime." She did not follow this with "little boy," and they weren't. The male movie icons of the time—Clark Gable, Jimmy Stewart, Gary Cooper, John Wayne, Gregory Peck, Cary Grant, and the rest—were all six footers. And even though the likes of Jimmy Cagney and Edward G. Robinson made it big, they were more in the way of character actors than romantic leading men. The current prominence of Al Pacino, Dustin Hoffman, and Michael J. Fox has not altered the perceptions ingrained in my youth.

Prejudice against short people also pervades the national scene. When a politician wishes to call up the image of a cherished leader from the past, it is always Washington, Jefferson, and Lincoln from whom they chose. True, these men were towering in more ways than in their physical presence, but think of the more moderately proportioned John Adams of Massachusetts, our second president, who contributed so much to the founding of our republic. And then consider the even more diminutive James Madison, our fourth president, who is rightly recognized as the "Father of the Constitution" and who also sponsored the Bill of Rights. When was the last time you heard their names called forth from a political podium? There are no monuments to short people in the District of Columbia!

When short men are mentioned at all, it is invariably in a bad light. They are often brought up as examples of troublemaking, ill-tempered, argumentative types: the likes of Napoleon, Kaiser Wilhelm, and Hitler, who were responsible for leading the world into wars and even worse.

In view of this, is there any advantage to being small? Well, for one thing, it is a lot easier to fit into modern airline seats. We also don't have to worry, upon entering a room, about bumping our heads on the doorway, nor crashing our skulls against low-hanging chandeliers. Clothes are usually easier to obtain without the need for size fourteen shoes and similarly gigantic suits and shirts. And although most women hate to have to look down upon their escorts, some rather statuesque types seem to adore us. Perhaps it is the mothering instinct, but whatever the origin of their urge, I am grateful for having been the occasional recipient of such Amazonian inclinations in the past.

There is another, a very special personal source of satisfaction with my size. In addition to being vertically challenged, despite comments to the contrary from my friends and family, I have always considered myself as "calorically confronted" (formerly "fat"), something I come by very legitimately. In genetic parlance, I can be considered homozygous for height as well as width: both my parents were short and boxlike, that symmetry interrupted only by the massive abdominal protuberances that, throughout their adult lives, blocked the sight line from head to toes. You might wonder how any source of comfort could be extracted from this self-image. I will explain.

To the outer world I bear the accoutrements of a physician and professor. In my heart of hearts, however, I possess the soul of a great tenor manqué. I cannot help but feel that had I only had a little more encouragement or courage in the past, I would have taken my rightful place among the operatic greats of this vocal register. Putting aside the sole exception, perhaps, of the towering Placido Domingo, all the great tenors—Enrico Caruso, Beniamino Gigli, Lauritz Melchior, Jussi Bjoerling, Ferruccio Tagliavini, Richard Tucker, Jan Peerce, Luciano Pavarotti—have been either short or fat or both. I find it reassuring that I fit the mold.

A small compensation, you might think, in view of the prevailing preferences in society. But, as a biological scientist, I have always had an additional source of consolation: the knowledge that although my length might have been shorter than that of others, my lifespan could be expected to be longer. Among mammals, I took note of how size was advantageous only to a point. While a mouse might live only three years and an elephant forty, humans, we know reach seventy, eighty, and more with regularity. Even within the same species, oversizing can be dangerous. Great Danes live only to the age of eight or nine while a lap dog can easily live one and a half to two times as long. Although I never thought of myself (metaphorically) as a Pekingese, such thoughts did give me an inner feeling of superiority over my sky-scraping friends.

Such conceptions of biological invulnerability have been fed by the likes of Tom Samaras, an engineer by profession, who has devoted over twenty years of his life to the study of bodily proportions and recently published his findings in a book.[2] According to Mr. Samaras and others he quotes who have conjointly analyzed the deaths of over eight thousand deceased people, it is better to be short. Whether you were a baseball player or a president; an anthropologist or a boxer; a veteran in San Diego or a resident of Cuyahoga County in Ohio; the shorter you were during life, the older you were likely to be at the conclusion of it.

Recently, however, a spate of new medical findings from what I consider more authoritarian sources have caused this aura of invincibility suddenly to fall about my ears. Up in Framingham, Massachusetts, where epidemiologists have been following the life courses of the inhabitants for over thirty-five years and relating health to a variety of factors, there comes a report that short stature is of no advantage whatsoever in men, and there may even be an increase in myocardial infarctions among shorter women.[3] The Physicians' Health Study, begun nationwide five years ago, indicates even worse news. Short doctors are more likely than tall ones to get coronary heart disease.[4] Meanwhile in Manitoba, Canada, nearly four thousand men who were considered fit for flight training back in 1948 and have been followed ever since, were found to have a statistically significant higher incidence of coronary disease related to short height, but "trends" toward an increase in overall mortality were also present.[5] To add insult to all this injury, the Norwegians now inform us that the shorter you are, the more likely you are to have a stroke.[6]

Such news would be devastating had not a new element intervened in my existence. In addition to being vertically challenged and calorically confronted, I turned sixty-five in 1994 and thus joined the ranks of those "experientially extended." I do not know that age has made me any wiser, but it has mellowed me a bit. Now, instead of wondering how long I am to live, I am more concerned with how well I have lived and am living at the moment. I am also becoming more concerned about how much I can contribute to the life quality of those about me, whatever their ages. In the final analysis, I believe *that* is the long and the short and all the rest of it.

Notes

1. Newman R. *Short People*. Little Criminals, Warner Bros. Records Inc. 1977.
2. Samaras TT. *The Truth about Your Height: Exploring the Myths and Realities of Human Size on Performance, Health, Pollution, and Survival*. San Diego, Calif.: Tecolote Publ, 1994.
3. Kannam JP, Levy D, Larson M, Wilson PWF. Short stature and risk for mortality and cardiovascular disease events. Circulation 1994; 90:2241–2247.
4. Hebert PR, Rich-Edwards JW, Manson J et al. Height and incidence of cardiovascular disease in male physicians. Circulation 1993; 88[part 1]:1437–1443.
5. Krahn AD, Manfreda J, Tate RB et al. Evidence that height is an independent risk factor for coronary artery disease (the Manitoba follow-up study). Am J Cardiol 1994; 74:398–399.
6. Njolstad I, Arnesen E, Lund-Larsen PG. Body height, cardiovascular risk factors, and risk of stroke in middle-aged men and women. Circulation 1996; 94:2877–2882.

20

On Chinese Restaurants, Prolapsing Heart Valves, and Other Medical Conundrums

MEDICINE HAS BEEN codified through centuries of observation and practice into groups of recognized diseases. These diseases have in turn been neatly grouped according to organ system and/or cause. Anything else with which we are confronted, unless it carries with it rather spectacular manifestations that simply cannot be ignored, is often dismissed as trivial, imaginary, or both. The "new" syndromes one reads about in the medical journals are often new only in the sense of being recently recognized officially, and they probably have been with us all along. However, once documented, they now become respectable and are legitimized by a name.

"Ah yes, Mrs. Jones. You are suffering from Acute Idiopathic Cervicospinal Myalgia. I was just reading about it the other day." (Translation: "Yes, I do believe that you really do experience sudden pains in the muscles of your neck and upper back although we have no idea of the cause—an idiopathic disease—but some respected authority has just reported ten cases of it in the latest edition of the *Annals of Internal Medicine*.") Functional hypoglycemia, mitral valve prolapse, and the Chinese Restaurant Syndrome all provide interesting examples of this.

The disorder now commonly called reactive or functional hypoglycemia was described originally in 1924 by Dr. Seale Smith of Birmingham, Alabama, but really began to catch on with the medical profession and the general public in the 1950s and 1960s.[1]

The theory was that postprandially some patients continued releasing insulin for hours, leading to drops in blood sugar levels and the manifestations of what might happen in any diabetic patient who has taken too much medication: an insulin reaction. These symptoms of palpitations, tingling, sweating, and nervousness also happen to describe an easily recognized psychiatric disorder, the typical "anxiety attack."

Inasmuch as anxiety attacks were recognized long before those of functional hypoglycemia became popularized, for many years patients in the latter category were simply classified by their physicians as slightly unbalanced mentally. With functional hypoglycemia achieving recognition, many were suddenly removed from the loony category (as they and their friends would have considered any mental derangement, no matter how minor to their psychiatrists) and comfortably installed in the realm of endocrinology. So comfortable for the patients and convenient for their doctors was "functional hypoglycemia" that, despite the fact that its validity as a common cause for such complaints has been challenged, it became the frequent diagnosis for many puzzling complaints about which patients and their doctors knew next to nothing as to cause or cure.

In more recent times, mitral valve prolapse has come to supersede functional hypoglycemia as a favorite unsubstantiated diagnosis in patients with nagging but unexplainable symptomatology. Although systolic bulging of the heart's mitral leaflets into the left atrium many be an accompaniment to other specific underlying heart diseases, it more often exists as an isolated phenomenon, rarely serious in nature, and often simply a normal variant with or without accompanying cardiac symptoms.

The mitral prolapse story has gone through several phases. For years mid-to-late systolic clicks, with or without accompanying murmurs auscultated in patients, were thought to be on an extracardiac basis. Then, thanks to three South Africans, the true cause of these phenomena became apparent. In 1961, J. V. Reid revived the concept that such clicks/murmurs arose in the heart, and then, through the clinical and angiographic study of large numbers of such patients, Drs. John Barlow and Wendy Pocock demonstrated the structural basis of such findings as originating in the mitral valve pattern of closure.[2]

It was the advent of echocardiography, however, that really put mitral prolapse on the diagnostic map, especially with the growing realization that angiographic prolapse studies were often subject to unacceptable variability in interpretation. Now with a simple, noninvasive technique, the diagnosis could be made with ease and better accuracy, especially in asymptomatic individuals or those with symptoms so minor as not to warrant cardiac catheterization to establish the diagnosis. In those patients with marked symptomatology suggestive of cardiac diseases—and they ran the gamut from palpitations to chest pain to fatigue and dizziness—we finally had an explanation for them and were able to convince our patients and ourselves that they were not simply imaginary. Furthermore, in almost all cases, we could assure the patients that, whatever the severity of their symptoms, their long-term outlook was excellent.

Then, gradually, confusion crept into the picture. First it became recognized that some symptomatic patients with mitral prolapse on echocardiography did not have the telltale click/murmurs when we listened to their hearts ("silent prolapse"). Even early on, with the ready availability and ease of cardiac ultrasound, prevalence studies in the general population revealed that many asymptomatic normals, especially young women, could demonstrate prolapse on echocardiography. From this we learned that mitral prolapse in many individuals was simply a normal variant. Finally, even the symptoms of mitral prolapse were deprived of their validity: studies of patients with and without mitral prolapse on echocardiography now suggest no difference in the incidence of most if not all of the symptoms we once considered typical of the syndrome.

Even the echocardiographic diagnosis of the prolapse pattern has undergone significant evolution. The earliest technique, M-mode, missed some cases which were then diagnosed by two-dimensional echocardiography, which came later. Then it was recognized that some of the M-mode and two-dimensional criteria had been too loosely applied, labelling many subjects as having prolapse when the diagnosis was based on simply a misinterpretation of a normal insertion pattern of the valve in certain views. As far as echocardiography is concerned, revisionism has reached such a point that in some quarters the criteria for prolapse have become so restrictive that even patients with obvious click-murmurs, whom most of us would accept as having prolapse, are now being denied the diagnosis by these investigators.

This is all very unfortunate because, in my view, we may do much more harm in underdiagnosing the condition than in granting it to patients in distress. One reason for this is that the prognosis is almost invariably excellent so we can be reassuring. Furthermore, the medication we prescribe for it, beta blockers, are often effective and reasonably safe. Their toning down of sympathetic discharges, whatever the cause, can be very helpful and, used only in times of stress, can sustain the patients quite effectively over the long haul. Many are the medical students I have helped through examination time with the judicious use of this diagnosis and treatment. The only drawback involves the medical insurance companies, which may increase their fees for those under the umbrella of this diagnosis.

The so-called Chinese Restaurant Syndrome provides a somewhat different kind of paradigm, one that struck quite close to home for me. For years, my sister-in-law complained about some ill-defined strange feelings each time she emerged from certain Chinese restaurants. These symptoms were experienced by no one else who accompanied her. As for the cause of her distress, we felt that she was an otherwise perfectly delightful, dependable, and reasonable member of the family and certainly entitled to one strange quirk.

Then, in April of 1968, a physician, appropriately named Kwok, wrote a letter to the editor of the *New England Journal of Medicine*.[3] In it he described a peculiar set of symptoms: a numbness or tingling at the back of the neck that extended over the shoulders and either down the arms or into the chest with a tight feeling about the temples. These symptoms only occurred fifteen to twenty minutes after he had completed eating dinner, usually Mandarin style, at one or two Chinese restaurants he frequented. He wondered if anyone else had knowledge of this disorder inasmuch as he had searched the medical literature for a description but to no avail.

In the ensuing weeks, almost a dozen physicians and medical students had their letters of reply printed in the journal. They had suffered similar symptoms under the same circumstances. One could almost read between the lines their sense of relief in finding a fellow sufferer and learning, at long last, that it was not "just in the head." Since then numerous more systematic forays into the mysteries of the syndrome have been made. Monosodium glutamate, used to enhance flavor, turns out to be the likely culprit. But, whatever the cause, it is now a perfectly respectable disorder with which to be afflicted.

The desire for symptomatic patients to be granted the sanctuary of a syndrome is probably matched only by the desire of certain intrepid or ambitious physicians to invent new ones to accommodate them. Failing this, they cannot resist the temptation of attempting publication of reports that can only be classified in the category of "Can you top this?" They may not raise the curtain on a new era of medical science, but at least they may raise a few eyebrows among the medical community.

One of the most common complaints among the general public, for example, is "gas," but it never really has received the kind of attention it might conceivably merit. An exception to this exclusion of serious scientific concern was made some years ago when studies of a flatulent patient were reported by a team at the University of Minnesota and published in the *New England Journal of Medicine* of all places. Before arriving at that fount of knowledge in the heart of Minneapolis, a twenty-eight-year-old man had consulted seven different physicians about his complaint. None of them had had anything to offer, and the patient had been reduced to keeping his own "flatographic" records. Over a one-year period, it was later determined by statistical analysis that he passed flatus an average of 34 ± 7.3 (standard deviation) times a day.

Under the meticulous observation of the Minnesota group, the patient was encouraged to continue his accurate record keeping. For their part, his physicians analyzed the gas and at one point even collected it to determine volume. (The methodology for the latter was not described, but it certainly provided an exercise for the imagination.) Finally, with the help of a lactose-free diet, the daily gas pass rate was reduced to 25 ± 8.2 SD, a significant drop from the thirty-four daily episodes he presented with. The authors were not totally immune to the potential responses of their august journal's readership. They concluded: "At present, the patient is assiduously testing a variety of foods in an attempt to develop a flatus-free palatable diet—thus far without a whiff of success."[4]

His experience with the University of Minnesota could not have been a total loss for the young man with the billowing bowels. There is always what the psychiatrists like to call "secondary gain" in conditions of adversity. During the course of his dietary manipulations, the effect of milk, two liters per day for two days, was observed. The result was an incredible daily flatus frequency of 141, with 70 passages within one four-hour period. This was submitted to the *Guinness Book of World Records* in hopeful anticipation.

Another investigator, this time from the Cleveland Clinic, has published an article entitled "Achoo Syndrome," which means exactly how it sounds.[5] He reported that four-of-twenty neurologists, questioned after a grand rounds conference held by their department, admitted to sneezing when gazing into a bright light. Since I have been doing this myself all my life, I took the trouble to question fifty randomly selected individuals passing me in the hallways of my own institution. After overcoming certain feelings of apprehension about my mental state, 12 or 24 percent of the total admitted to a similar pattern of photic response. Now, just to save you countless sleepless nights pondering the meaning of all this, the author of this epic-making discovery has deduced that the cause lies not in our stars, Horatio, but in our genes. Believe it or not, the photic reflex may actually be caused by an autosomal dominant gene with variable expressivity.

A team of researchers from Boston's Brigham-Women's Hospital have demonstrated even more enviable chutzpah in their description of two cases of "giggle incontinence."[6] Any of us who has ever heard the expression "I laughed so hard the tears ran down my leg" can certainly appreciate that one!

And for all you philanderers out there, a ready source of comfort has been on tap for years in another letter to the *New England Journal of Medicine*. It describes sexual intercourse and transient global amnesia in two patients.[7] The next time your wife confronts you, simply reply "What secretary? What intercourse?" and refer her to the April 12, 1979, issue.

What other fascinating ailments are awaiting the attention of some totally honest but foolhardy physician? The "Chronic Fatigue Syndrome" certainly looms on the horizon as a likely contender, whatever its relationship to the Epstein-Barr virus.[8] Certainly there are millions of us who are chronically fatigued and would love to be able to blame it on some "bug." For my part, however, since the strictly scholarly category is disclaimed here, there is no hesitation in putting forth my own prime candidate: The Cine-Cephalgia Galoshes Syndrome.

As a child en route to a Saturday movie matinee on a rainy afternoon, I was frequently admonished by my mother to remove my galoshes in the theater or else suffer a severe headache and premature blindness. To this day the neglect of this ritual in a darkened motion-picture house results in a troublesome pain behind the eyes and a slight blurring of vision. One day, almost laughingly I recounted this story to a friend and his mother. The latter quickly replied, "Of course, everybody knows that!" We now await a high-powered team of experts from the National Institutes of Health to report on the effects of rubber-enclosed extremities on reflex pathways between the sensory receptors of the toes and certain regions of the brain.

Notes

1. Hofeldt FD. Reactive hypoglycemia. Metabolism 1975; 24:1193–1208.
2. Barlow JB and Pocock WA. The problem of non-ejection systolic clicks and associated mitral systolic murmurs: Emphasis on the billowing mitral leaflet syndrome. Am Heart J 1975; 90:636–655.
3. Kwok RHM. Chinese restaurant syndrome. N Engl J Med 1968; 278:796.
4. Levitt MD, Lasser RB, Schwartz JS, Bond JH. Studies of a flatulent patient. N Engl J Med 1976; 295:260–262.

5. Morris HH III. Achoo syndrome. Cleveland Clin J Med 1987; 54:431–433.
6. Rogers MP, Gittes RF, Dawson DM, Reich P. Giggle incontinence. JAMA 1982; 247:1446.
7. Mayeux R. Sexual intercourse and transient global amnesia. N Engl J Med 1979; 300:864.
8. Holmes GP et al. Chronic fatigue syndrome: A working case definition. Ann Intern Med 1988; 108:387.

21

So, You Want to Be a Doctor?

THERE ARE A number of reasons arguing against taking up the study of medicine in the nineties and beyond. Once one of the last bastions of individualism in an increasingly regimented society, American medicine has seen its autonomy eaten away by federal and state bureaucracies; we have been battered by the development of HMOs and the like; and our remains are often prey to legalistic sharks in a sea of litigation.

We may be producing too many doctors, with future employment opportunities severely diminishing. For those whose interest in medicine may be spurred primarily by an aptitude for investigation, research funds are dwindling with our growing preoccupation with the national debt and a Congress intent on lowering taxes whatever the cost to many of our most worthy federal programs. Potential medical school applicants with a financial bent might also be interested to learn that, except for procedure-based specialists (the numbers of which are currently being severely restricted), potential medical doctors would have a much better return on their investment over a lifetime of employment if they chose a career in business, law, or even dentistry.[1]

There is only one argument to counter all these negative considerations: the study and practice of medicine remains one of the most interesting and gratifying career pursuits that anyone could desire, at least in the opinion of this writer, who has been at it for so long and lived through so many changes.

Over the years, many aspirants and their families have contacted me for advice along these lines, but never as many as I would hope to have reached. Having followed such a long and tortuous path to medicine myself, I have always wanted to impart to others the knowledge I have gained along the way as an applicant, student, medical school faculty member, and, later, admissions committee chairperson. For those who are not discouraged by the negative elements affecting medicine that seem so often to predominate in the news, in other words, for those who decide to pursue a medical career, the sooner you can focus on this goal the better, best of all as a high school senior.

First of all, try to gain admission to the best *undergraduate* college of your choice, even if you have to scrub floors to pay your way through it. "Best" does not equate with "biggest." Oftentimes it is the smaller school, the one where you can obtain more personal attention, that will help you most in reaching your goal. There are many prestigious smaller schools; try to find out which they are and which ones might be for you. The quality of the school that you choose, large or small, will be uppermost in the minds of medical school admissions committees and, all else being equal between two applicants, they will choose the one from the better school. In addition, attempt to find out from each school to which you apply how many premedical students have attended there and what percentage of success they have had in placing their premed students in medical school. They all have that information, and if they say they do not, they are not worth applying to in the first place.

Your first stop, after your parents, will be the guidance counselor at your high school. Be wary. Some high schools take pride in this and place superb people in such positions. At other high schools it turns out that the most inept member of the staff is in charge of this and has usually held on to the position through decades of ineptitude. You will probably know within the first year of your high school career about the reputation of the guidance office. If there is any doubt about this, find out the percentage of college admissions from your school's graduating classes and to which colleges the seniors over the last few years have been admitted. If the answer comes back in the "number of admissions" to prestigious schools rather than the number of students accepted, this is misleading. A single student, the top in the class, being admitted to five Ivy League schools is not the same as five different students heading in that direction. Finally, if the guidance counselor is hopeless and your parents are not informed about higher education opportunities, seek other adults among their acquaintance or religious affiliation (e.g., church membership) who might provide guidance.

Once in college, you must recognize that your primary task is to get good grades, especially in the sciences. There is a movement afoot among medical schools (I almost wrote "fad") to downplay the traditional scientific training in college, and some schools have even cut such requirements to the bare bone. I believe this trend will pass, especially as we become more and more aware of how American education in mathematics and science has fallen behind our world competitors and how we must do something to correct this imbalance. There is a lot that can be said for extracurricular activity; this can help make you a more "well-rounded person." But it will help your chances for medical school acceptance only if your scholastic record is up to the mark.

If you wish to enhance your chances for acceptance through extracurricular activity, use your weekends and vacation time to advantage. This can start as early as high school. Research positions, assisting medical school faculty in their projects, are the most desirable type of work to find, but this is often difficult, and more so the younger and more inexperienced you are. For the high school and college student though, there is the opportunity to work on emergency squads and in hospitals where volunteers are always wanted or hard to fill low-paying positions are often available.

What happens when you reach your senior year in college and are about to begin the application process? If you are an A student or close to it, there is nothing to worry about. If you do not get an acceptance to a highly prestigious school, you may have several offers from others, all good places to train, with scholarships more likely to be available for the bright if not exceptional student. Fortunately, the restrictive practices against Jews and Catholics should no longer be a problem if one meets the standards. As for disadvantaged minority group members, there may be special programs set up for such groups in certain medical schools. Make it your business to learn where if you fall into this category.

Demographics are an important consideration for all medical school applicants. The ratio of applicants to acceptances will vary from state to state. Almost all states have at least one state-supported school, and in these the overwhelming number of acceptances go to state residents. Private schools are not obligated to favor state residents and infrequently do. Extreme examples are Arizona, a state school where, in 1996, 100 percent of the entrants were state residents, and Harvard, where only 15.9 percent fell into this category. The Association of American Colleges' Section for Student Services in Washington, D.C., prepares a report on applicants, matriculants, and graduates that you may send away for to calculate the odds as they apply to you. Another valuable source of information is the medical education issue of the *Journal of the American Medical Association*, usually published in September of each year. In addition to listing all the U.S. schools, it includes information regarding the number of in-state and out-of-state admissions, and other critical information, not least of which is the tuition costs at each school. Most private schools are fairly expensive, while a number of state schools may charge only a fraction of the typical private school tuition. In an era when our seniors are often graduating with loan debts amounting to fifty or one hundred thousand dollars, this is an important consideration. Copies of the *Journal of the American Medical Association* can be found in almost any physician's office, the local county medical library, or other public libraries as well as medical schools.

Another point to keep in mind is, if, after a year or two of college, you are not doing as well as you think you need to in order to attend a medical school in your own state, and there is another state where you would stand a better chance as a resident, look into the possibility of switching schools and establishing residency there to make yourself eligible.

What is the importance of the Medical College Admission Test (MCAT) in determining your fate? It is generally agreed among admissions officers that this is definitely secondary to your grade point average, which reflects your performance over a three to four year period rather than just how well you did on a couple of days of examination when you may not have been at your best. I do have the impression, however, that, if your chances for admission are borderline, an impressive showing on these examinations might put you over the hump. Having said that, I am obliged to address the question of preparatory courses for taking these tests. It is probably true that a number of these courses can raise scores a few percentage points, and for the student in the gray zone of acceptance, such considerations might apply.

What about recommendations? Your college recommendation is important along with the adviser's ability to place a large number of his premedical students.

Recommendations from politicians are usually worthless. Being a member of "a fine family" that, itself, might only vaguely be known to the politico, will have no influence on any admissions committee. Knowing someone on the admissions committee, paradoxically, might help you the least. In today's moral climate, most committee members consider themselves pretty independent and above reproach. Any attempt of one admissions committee member to influence the others on a candidate of his choice is usually a guarantee of that applicant's rejection. Only a full-time faculty member, usually not a member of the committee and one for whom you have done some work, can favorably influence your application. Here a letter describing your intelligence, industry, and reliability can really have an effect.

Many doctors in the community have clinical appointments to medical schools and are described as "professors at the medical school" by their patients. The number of hours they actually devote to the school varies widely and often their connection with such institutions is only quite peripheral. It is unlikely that the overwhelming majority have any influence on admissions either at the school at which they volunteer or their alma maters. Even the days when deans, for example, routinely had the courtesy extended to them of placing one or two students in each freshman class are largely over, especially at state-supported institutions where strictly ethical practices are usually adhered to. At our own school, each applicant is graded by the various members of the admissions committee, and the composite score listed in order for each year. Admissions are offered in turn, going down the list until a class is filled. From what I have been able to gather from conversations with others, similar processes of admission are in place at most other public schools although I suspect that at private institutions there may be more latitude for special decision making.

Given all of the above, what are your chances? Since about two-thirds of all those applying to American medical schools will fail to gain admission on their first try, unless you have managed to achieve an outstanding undergraduate record, statistically you are more likely than not to be rejected rather than accepted. What do you do then?

There is nothing more disheartening than searching the mailbox each morning for almost a year in search of an acceptance, only to find no news or bad news. Each letter of rejection is likely to lower your own self-esteem another notch so that at the end of the process you might find yourself wondering whether or not you should ever have embarked on such a career choice in the first place. For some this may indeed have represented an overambitious miscalculation. But for many it should rather be looked upon as only the first stop along the way to achieving your life's ambition. You should recognize that although the first wave of applicants to be accepted, perhaps 20 or 30 percent of the total, were clearly superior to the rest, the differences between successive groups of those accepted become increasingly imperceptible. I know of one southwestern medical school where, following completion of the initial admissions process, the number of slots in the freshman class was expanded by twenty or thirty places. The academic performance of this additional group enrolled was subsequently compared with that of the equal number admitted before them, and there were no differences found.

Therefore, if you determine that your plans were not completely off the mark, the first thing to do is to review the strategy of the previous year and see where you might improve the second time around. Did you apply to *enough* schools? Did you apply to the *right* schools, those where you stood the best chance of gaining admission? On your next try do not feel that an initial rejection will be held against you. A second attempt is more likely to be looked upon as a sign of perseverance and seriousness of purpose rather than as a strike against you.

How did you do on your MCATs? If you perceive that these constituted a mark against you, you should probably take them again and not hesitate to enroll in one of the preparatory courses offered to insure that your grades the second time around will be improved.

Following an initial rejection of applications to medical school, some might be tempted to enter one of the fields of allied health that are proving increasingly attractive. Physicians assistants, especially, will assume a prominent role in the cost conscious operation of our hospitals and medical practices in the coming years. However the number of places in such training programs are limited and may, in certain instances, be even more competitive than medical school admissions. And, in the final analysis, if it is a doctor you really wish to become, even if you do enter one of these fields, there is always likely to be a feeling of emptiness and failure when you have decided upon accepting anything less than this, especially when you are placed in contact with doctors each day of your working life. There are other options.

One of these is the study of osteopathy. You might consider applying to one or more of these schools concurrently with your first try at medicine or in the year following an unsuccessful application. Schools of osteopathy are usually not as competitive as medical schools, offer good training, and if the student is so inclined, allow for a later opportunity during the residency period to switch into the medical mainstream. Many D.O.'s (doctors of osteopathy), especially those becoming interested in subspecialty training, are welcome in M.D. residency programs where such opportunities are usually much more developed than in hospitals run by osteopaths. (Please do not confuse osteopathy with chiropractic.)

Another option, as you undergo another year or two of the admissions process, is to obtain a position as a research assistant at the medical school of your choice. The time you spend in the company of faculty there will give them a chance to become acquainted with you and, when the time comes, give you a strong and meaningful recommendation (provided, of course, you merit it). An equally good or possibly even better option is to enroll in a graduate program in one of the biological sciences at a medical complex (e.g., anatomy, biochemistry, physiology, pharmacology). This may eventually lead you into a Ph.D.-M.D. program or a simple direct transfer into medical school with credits given you for the basic science portion you have completed. I have observed a number of students making these kinds of transition from research and graduate positions in biological science into medical school at our own institution and am sure it is not uncommon elsewhere.

Are foreign medical schools an option? Those of us raised in the American medical educational system, especially since World War II, have always looked upon much foreign-based medical training with something of a jaundiced eye. The educational programs and facilities at many of these institutions were often considered substandard (see Greetings chapter). However, over time, as I have come in contact with house staff who have emerged from such schools and managed to work their way into stateside medical residency programs, I have often been impressed with the high quality of many of these young men and women. They are often out to prove something about their ability, and more often than not, they seem to succeed. Remember, you don't have to be a genius to be a good doctor. All the intelligence in the world will avail nothing to a doctor's patients unless that physician is fully dedicated to their welfare. Many foreign medical graduates, I find, fulfill this critical requirement.

Although I have no personal problem with this, my views may not be shared by others in similar positions. A large part of our attitude toward foreign medical graduates depends upon our perception of a need for them. Predicting whether or not there will be an excess or shortage of physicians twenty years hence is a notoriously difficult task to perform with any degree of accuracy or assurance. The consensus at present, however, is that there will be a future surplus of physicians in general and that there is undoubtedly a surplus of most medical specialists and subspecialists at present. In order to reduce the number of physicians in general, it is most effective to reduce the number of those in residency training, the only conduit into professional practice that exists for medical graduates. The Council on Graduate Medical Education[2] and the Physician Payment Review Commission[3] have both recommended that the federal government limit the number of entry-level residency positions in the United States to 110 percent of the number of U.S. medical school graduates. The Clinton administration has come out in support of this.

The primary target of such a reduction in training places will be in the foreign medical schools, about which a recent report from the U.S. General

Accounting Office provides a number of important findings.[4] It turns out, as of 1990–1991, about 83 percent of U.S. nationals attending foreign medical schools were matriculated in unapproved programs. In 1994, graduates of U.S. medical schools accounted for 17,500 first year residency slots. An additional 6,750 were filled by foreign medical school graduates of whom 17 percent were U.S. citizens. Although it is likely that non-U.S. foreign medical graduates will be the first to suffer the initial curtailment on admission to hospital residencies here, if and when they go into full effect, foreign-trained U.S. citizens may be affected as well.

For those who ultimately intend to go this route despite the current uncertainties, recent publications for the guidance of applicants and hospital program directors as well have appeared.[5] Finally, before you enroll in a foreign medical school, determine where they place their students for hospital training, determine if the hospitals plan to continue this association, check the attitudes of your own state medical boards, and be sure to have discussions with recent graduates of the school to determine how they fared.

Good luck to you all!

Notes

1. Weeks WA, Wallace AE, Wallace MM, Welch HG. A comparison of the educational costs and incomes of physicians and other professionals. New Engl J Med 1994; 330:1280–1286.

2. Council on Graduate Medical Education. Third report: Improving access to health care through physician workforce reform: Directions for the twenty-first century. Washington, D.C.: Department of Health and Human Services, 1992.

3. Annual Report to Congress. Washington, D.C.: Physician Payment Review Commission, 1993.

4. Student Loans: Millions Loaned Inappropriately to U.S. Nationals at Foreign Medical Schools (General Accounting Office, HEHS-94-28, January 1994).

5. *International Medical Graduates in U.S. Hospitals: A Guide for Program Directors and Applicants.* Khan FA and Smith LG eds. Philadelphia, Pa.: American Coll Physicians, 1995; Ball LB. *The International Medical Graduates' Guide to U.S. Medicine.* Tucson, Ariz.: Galen Press, 1995.

22

While the Getting's Good

My wife and I have a long-standing running joke about a joke. The joke, the original one, concerns an increasingly wealthy widow who is in the process of burying her third well-heeled husband who has died under unusual circumstances. At the funeral she is approached by an uninhibited guest whose curiosity has gotten the better of him. He asks, "Isn't it strange that your first two husbands died from eating poisonous mushrooms while this one fell off a high building?"

"Well you see," the black widow explains, "the last one didn't like mushrooms."

Both of us physicians, my wife and I have observed at close hand the ravages that advancing age and disease can wreak upon patients. We are even more closely tuned in to the effects of these on ourselves and our colleagues. As a full-time faculty member whose practice is primarily limited to hospital work, I am especially concerned with the aging physician within these settings in particular. My wife and I have agreed to keep a watchful eye on each other, and when one of us is beginning to prove an embarrassment to himself or herself or, worse, a danger to the patients, we have promised to do something about it. Something short of marital mayhem, of course, but "passing the poisonous mushrooms" is our shorthand for the application of such measures for universal protection.

Having observed others falter in my time, the older I get, the more often I think of when the time will come when I too will begin to operate without "hitting on all cylinders" all the time.

Among all the medical specialties, it is in surgery, which Harvard's Francis Moore once described as "an athletic event," that can provide the most striking examples of what tragedies might befall patients and surgeons alike when the latter continue operating beyond the limits of their diminished capabilities. Stories of surgical chiefs rushing to the operating room to "bail out" an aging colleague who has blundered are not uncommon. However, even greater problems may arise when it is the chief, himself, who has hung on too long and cannot be budged from his position of authority.

The most dramatic of these accounts involved that of the great German surgeon, Ferdinand Sauerbruch (1875–1951), who at twenty-nine years of age in 1904 was the first to devise a method to operate safely on the contents of the chest and thus ushered in the era of lung, esophageal, and heart surgery. From such auspicious beginnings, Sauerbruch ascended from one prestigious post to another, finally achieving the pinnacle as chief of the surgical clinic at Berlin's Charité Hospital where he served for the last two decades of his career.

By 1949, however, Sauerbruch began to show distinct signs of what was then called "senile cerebral sclerosis" and what we would now label as Alzheimer's disease. In *The Dismissal*, Jurgen Thorwald's detailed account of Sauerbruch's decline and fall, Thorwald describes one particularly hair-raising episode that has been etched on my memory.

A governmental official was visiting Sauerbruch in his office when an assistant, white gowned and gloved, appeared at the doorway to report on a patient whom he had been preparing in the operating room for Sauerbruch. He announced that, upon exposing the brain, he had found the tumor they anticipated to be too advanced for surgical intervention; the patient was inoperable. Sauerbruch, enraged, rushed out of the office to the operating suite and returned less than a quarter of an hour later still growling about the incompetence of his assistants. In his hands he held a pulpy pink mass which he held out for the horrified visitor's inspection. Without even scrubbing or gowning up, Sauerbruch had plucked the tumor from the brain with his bare hands.

Incredibly, following such bizarre behavior, Sauerbruch continued to operate at the Charité for some months and then, following his forced resignation, at a private clinic and even at his home before his death in 1951.

Nonsurgical tales of such malfeasance are much less dramatic but still impressive enough for those involved in such care to be wary of practitioners who attempt continuing beyond the point when they can still function effectively. It should not be surprising to see relatively young physicians bemoaning the spectacle of aging colleagues vainly attempting to persist beyond their span of useful service. What has impressed me, however, are the number of preeminent physicians, well into their maturity, who have been the most forceful in expressing these sentiments.

Johns Hopkins' William Osler (1849–1919) is remembered as one of our most distinguished and revered internists and is often quoted in regard to this question. Among a series of talks he delivered, in one he called "The Fixed Period" he commented upon "the comparative uselessness of men above forty years of age" and the uselessness of men above sixty. In more recent times, the wittily pungent Sir George Pickering (1904–1980) of Oxford, despairing over the inability of older physicians to accept new ideas, once wrote "Where there is death there is hope."

One of my own most admired mentors, cardiologist William Dock (1898–1990), was unremitting in his condemnation of those doctors who simply held on too long and repeatedly expressed his admiration for those who had departed from practice even before the question of diminishing capacities could be raised. He loved to recall that Hippocrates identified fifty-six as the beginning of senility, along with echoing Osler's sentiments expressed above. "Here's your coat. What's your hurry?" was his motto, and with great gusto he would tell the joke about the professor who returned home to inform his grandson that he had just been made emeritus.

"I know Latin," the boy responded, "E means you're out, and 'meritus' means you God damned well deserve it."

As someone who started medical school a few years later than my classmates, I always felt that I had some catching up to do and have been a little defensive about premature elimination of faculty just because they happen to reach a certain age. I once pointed out to Dock that chronological age and biological age are often at odds with one another; that there are those who at sixty may act as if they were eighty while, conversely, there were some in their eighties who had the vim and vigor of fifty-year-olds. Dock, who certainly fell into the latter category, didn't hesitate to reply, "That may be so, but if you are the subject under discussion you have no idea which one you are. So just get out and the sooner the better."

Getting out, or rather getting others to get out, seems to be a high priority among many academic institutions today. Unless a senior physician is still the recipient of a large federal grant with many overhead dollars pouring into the university coffers, or with a large faculty practice that accomplishes the same goal, they want him or her out pronto.

I suppose it is too much to expect that, as in times past, an aging faculty member who has devoted twenty, thirty, forty years of his life to a university, might be granted a little space and a few tasks to perform in his final years. I suppose that all this might fit under the heading of "sentimental hogwash" to the members of these multilayered, overstaffed, and overstuffed administrations (from the faculty's viewpoint) who now look upon themselves as simply being efficient businessmen in the best tradition of corporate executives. But if it is simply the bottom line on which they are focused, I suggest that their vision might be tunneled.

The days when you can hire two bright young assistant professors for the price of one full professor are gone, at least as this pertains to many parts of present-day medicine. With salary increases over the years lagging behind inflation and the demands of the current marketplace, a talented young person at the assistant professor level might demand as much or even more than a tenured full professor who has been on the faculty for several decades. This is undoubtedly true for some of the surgical specialties as well as the procedure-oriented specialties within departments of internal medicine and others.

Many senior physicians would be happy to go on a half-time status, but this often seems unacceptable to administrations making such decisions. Instead, they dangle early retirement packages as inducements for such faculty to leave. However, a year's salary or even a bit more to someone sixty years of age with a life expectancy of eighty or more is hardly reassuring, and thus many senior faculty who would gladly reduce their working hours at their institutions and thus make room for additional new blood are dissuaded from such a course by these realities. The end result of this situation seems to be that, thanks to increasing legislation against age discrimination, many faculty as well as other employees may be staying on longer than even they originally intended.

To this observer, it seems that administrations of medical schools and perhaps other institutions, in their misguided zeal for cost cutting and/or updating of their faculty, are overlooking a valuable resource represented by older faculty and staff members.

Those among this group with past research experience can serve as useful guides to junior faculty just beginning their careers. For the more clinically oriented faculty, their value might lie in filling in the clinical responsibilities for their juniors who are more intent on making their mark in research and obtaining funding for it in the first place. Such senior faculty, wise in the way of hospital and school committee work, can also occupy these time consuming slots to permit the others to proceed with their scientific careers unimpeded. In certain departments that are shorthanded and immediately in difficulty because one of their members is out with illness, on vacation, or possibly on sabbatical, the availability of a part-timer to fill in can be invaluable.

Finally, one of the greatest deficiencies of our current medical educational system lies in its inability to provide bedside teaching of the art of medicine to medical students and house staff. Who might be better qualified than those physicians who have already filled their lives with such experiences?

All these arguments will, I am quite sure, fall on deaf ears in the areas where they might do the most good. I will probably be looked upon as just another of those aging physicians trying to justify his own existence as he nears the end of his professional rope. Actually, most of the time I feel as if I were forty; I look into the mirror and am vain enough to think I could pass for fifty; the truth is I am irrevocably past sixty. However, I still feel that I am performing more work than many in my professional acquaintance half my age. I am torn between such strong personal convictions and the admonitions of Osler, Hippocrates, and Dock.

I would much rather jump than be pushed and in this respect I recall another great physician, Arthur L. Bloomfield of Stanford who, following his retirement as chairman of medicine, continued to make hospital teaching rounds at the University of California hospitals in San Francisco when he was in his seventies. I was fortunate enough to have Dr. Bloomfield as my attending physician when, in 1960, I was a first year medical resident at the Fort Miley Veterans Administration Hospital there. To me he always seemed "right on the button," and in his more expansive moods, when he began to give us the perspective of his broad historical view of medicine, it was a revelation.

I learned later that each year he offered his resignation to the chief of staff, not wishing to outstay his welcome. I would hope that, when the time comes, I might have the same confidence in my ability to do the same, but I probably will not take this route for myself. Given my often prickly and outspoken nature, I am sure the powers that be would jump at the chance to dump me and regret only that I had not made the offer ten or fifteen years earlier. More likely I will take my cue from Dr. Willem J. Kolff, the developer of the first practical artificial kidney among his many other contributions to the field of artificial organs. When I interviewed him about fifteen years ago, he was in his seventies, and the last time I checked, he was still active in medical research. I had asked him how long he expected to go on. He replied that he would continue to work as long as he was having fun.

Me too—unless the poisonous mushrooms get me first.

(Postscript: Three years after writing this article, the author resigned his full-time medical school position. It was time to move on.)

Index

Index

Achoo Syndrome, 126
affirmative action: at New Jersey Medical School, 13–15; *University of California v. Bakke*, 12–13
aging doctors: Dock on, 139; medical school policies, 139–40; Osler on, 138–39; and productivity, 139; roles for, 140–41
anemia: sickle cell, 60; in tuberculosis, 39–40
antisemitism: and medical school admissions 5–9; and professional advancement, 7, 11
Asian-Americans and higher education, 16; at New Jersey Medical School, 57, 107
Auerbach, Oscar, 39–40

Bakke, Allan P. *See* affirmative action: *University of California v. Bakke*
Banting, Frederick, 20
Bean, William Bennett, 34–35
Beaumont, William: and Alexis St. Martin, 79–80; observations on gastric physiology, 80
Best, Charles H., 20
Bloomfield, Arthur L., 41, 141
books: influence on choosing medical career, 55–59
Braverman, Morris: and anemia of tuberculosis, 40
Brooks, Chandler McCuskey, 10
Burt, Cyril, 47–48
Burwell, C. Sidney, 45

Campylobacter. *See* Heliobacter pylori
cancer. *See* infection and cancer
Carini, Antonio, 30–33
Carrel, Alexis, 18
Chagas, Carlos, 30–32
Chinese Restaurant Syndrome, 125
Chronic Fatigue Syndrome, 127
Comroe, Julius H., Jr., 45

Conversations in Medicine (Weisse): Kornberg interview, 6, 11
coronary heart disease: and diet, 52; and exercise, 51; and height, 120–21; and type A personality, 52
Cotzias, George, 48
Cruz, Oswaldo, 30–32

Darsee, John, 47
Dismissal, The (Thorwald), 138
Dock, William: on aging, 139
dogs: use in medical research, 65–68
Double Helix, The (Watson), 50
Dubos, René, 38

Experiments and Observations on the Gastric Juice and the Physiology of Digestion (Beaumont), 79–80

Fibiger, Johannes, 47; Nobel Award in Physiology and Medicine (1926), 74; and Spiroptera carcinoma, 73–75, 83
financial rewards: according to medical specialty, 71–72; physicians vs. others, 129
Fishbein, Morris, 7
"Fixed Period, The" (Osler), 138–39
flatulence, 125–26
For the Love of Enzymes (Kornberg), 62
Friedman, Meyer, 52, 103

Gajdusek, D. Carleton, 30
giggle incontinence, 127
Good, Robert A., 48

height: and coronary heart disease, 120–21; and longevity, 120; and stroke, 121
Helicobacter pylori: culturing of, 77–78; and

gastritis/peptic ulcer, 76–81; and neoplasia, 81–82; presence in stomach, 76
Herrick, James B., 60–61
Holmes, Oliver Wendell, 40, 43–44
hypoglycemia, functional, 122–23

infection and cancer, 82–83; H. pylori and cancer, 81–82
Internal Revenue Service, 97–102

Johns Hopkins University, 11; Blalock at, 19; Halsted at, 19; Taussig at, 19; Wintrobe at, 11
Joining the Club: A History of Jews and Yale (Oren), 5

Kean, Benjamin, 31
Keys, Ancel, 52
Knopf, Sigard Adolphus, 42–43
Koch, Robert, 41–42
Koch's postulates, 42; in proof of H. pylori and gastritis, 81
Kornberg, Arthur, 6; autobiography, 62
Krebs, Sir Hans A.: and citric acid cycle, 61

Laennec, Theophile, 38–39
Linnaeus, 30
Ludwig, Karl, 18

males and mating behavior, 26–28
Marshall, Barry, 73, 76–79; collaboration with Warren, 76–79; letter to Lancet, 79; self experimentation with H. pylori, 81
McLeod, John R., 20
medical education: among children of physicians, 88–91; cost of, 87; financial rewards of, 71–72
medical school admission: advice to applicants, 129–36; and antisemitism, 5–9; and blacks, 7, 13–16; and geography, 4, 131–32; for World War II Veterans, 4
medical school applicants: advice to, 129–36; changing numbers, 90
mitral valve prolapse, 123–25

names: foreign in the United States, 104–6; misspelling of, 103
New Jersey Medical School: affirmative action at, 13–15
Newton, Isaac, 18
Nobel Prize in Physiology and Medicine: for citric acid (Krebs) cycle, 61; for discovery of insulin, 20; for discovery of streptomycin, 20, 38; for Spiroptera carcinoma, 47, 73–75

Osler, William: on aging and productivity, 92–94, 138–39; biography of, 33–34; on keeping up to date, 61; use of "white scourge," 39

peptic ulcer and Helicobacter pylori, 79–81
Pneumocystis carinii: and AIDS, 29; discovery of, 31–32; naming of, 32

race: in medical publication, 110; and medical school admissions (N.J.), 11–13; and political correctness, 107–9
Retrospectroscope: Insights into Medical Discovery (Comroe), 45
Rous, Peyton, 47, 75

Sauerbruch, Ferdinand, 138
Schatz, Albert, 20, 38
Seton Hall College of Medicine. *See* New Jersey Medical School
SI Units: arguments against, 114, 116; arguments for, 114; derivation, 114
Sokolof, Leon, 8–9
Stunkard, Horace W., 2–3
Summerlin, William, 48

Truth About Your Height: Exploring The Myths and Realities of Human Size on Performance, Health, Pollution and Survival, The (Samaras), 120
tuberculosis: in ancient Greece, 37–38; anemia in, 40; *Bargaining for Life* (Bates), 41; clinical course, 37–38; *Forgotten Plague, The* (Ryan), 41; *Historical Chronology of Tuberculosis, An* (Burke), 38; *Living in the Shadow of Death* (Rothman), 42; pathology of, 38–39; "white" and, 38; *White Plague, The* (Dubos), 38
Tuchman, Barbara, 33

University of Utah School of Medicine: early cardiology research of author at, 21–23; Wintrobe at, 11

Villemin, J. A., 41
von Linné, Carl. *See* Linnaeus

Waksman, Selman, 20; and Nobel Prize, 20; use of "white plague," 38

Wangensteen, Owen H., 19
Warren, J. Robin, 76–79; letter to Lancet, 79
Weinstein, Louis, 7
white plague. *See* tuberculosis

Who Goes First? (Altman), 68
Wiggers, Carl J., 19
Winternitz, Milton, 7
Wintrobe, Maxwell M., 11, 19

Allen B. Weisse, M.D., is a practicing cardiologist and professor of medicine at the New Jersey College of Medicine in Newark. Among his previously published books are *The Man's Guide to Good Health*; *Medical Odysseys*; *Medicine: The State of the Art*, coauthored with Charles Mangel; and the award-winning *Conversations in Medicine*, an oral history of interviews with outstanding medical scientists.